SOVIET
MILITARY
PSYCHIATRY

OTHER BOOKS BY RICHARD A. GABRIEL

Military Incompetence: Why the US Military Doesn't Win

Operation Peace for Galilee: The Israeli-PLO War in Lebanon

The Antagonists: A Comparative Combat Assessment of the Soviet and American Soldier

The Mind of the Soviet Fighting Man

To Serve With Honor: A Treatise on Military Ethics and the Way of the Soldier

Fighting Armies: NATO and the Warsaw Pact

Fighting Armies: Antagonists of the Middle East

Fighting Armies: Third World Armies

The New Red Legions: An Attitudinal Portrait of the Soviet Soldier

The New Red Legions: A Survey Data Sourcebook

Crisis in Command: Mismanagement in the US Army

Managers and Gladiators: Directions of Change in the US Army

Ethnic Groups in America

Program Evaluation: A Social Science Approach

The Ethnic Factor in the Urban Polity

The Environment: Critical Factors in Strategy Development

SOVIET MILITARY PSYCHIATRY

The Theory and Practice of Coping with Battle Stress

RICHARD A. GABRIEL

CONTRIBUTIONS IN MILITARY STUDIES, NUMBER 53

GREENWOOD PRESS
NEW YORK • WESTPORT, CONNECTICUT • LONDON

Library of Congress Cataloging-in-Publication Data

Gabriel, Richard A.
  Soviet military psychiatry

  (Contributions in military studies, ISSN 0883–6884;
no. 53)
  Bibliography: p.
  Includes index.
  1. Psychiatry, Military. 2. Combat—Psychological
aspects. 3. Soviet Union—Armed Forces—Medical care.
I. Title. II. Series.
UH6295.S65G33 1986   616.85′212   85–24795
ISBN 0–313–25225–4 (lib. bdg. : alk. paper)

Copyright © 1986 by Richard A. Gabriel

All rights reserved. No portion of this book may be
reproduced, by any process or technique, without the
express written consent of the publisher.

Library of Congress Catalog Card Number: 85–24795
ISBN: 0–313–25225–4
ISSN: 0883–6884

First published in 1986

Greenwood Press, Inc.
88 Post Road West
Westport, Connecticut 06881

Printed in the United States of America

∞

The paper used in this book complies with the
Permanent Paper Standard issued by the National
Information Standards Organization (Z39.48–1984).

10 9 8 7 6 5 4 3 2 1

For my daughters, Christine and Leah.
Life is full of trials; may you always
be found innocent... or, at least, not
guilty.

Discipline keeps enemies face-to-face a little longer, but cannot supplant the instinct of self-preservation, and the sense of fear that goes with it. Fear! There are officers and soldiers who do not know it, but they are people of rare grit. The mass shudders; because you cannot suppress the flesh.

—Ardant Du Picq, 1862

Contents

Tables	ix
Preface	xi
Acknowledgments	xv
1. Origins of Soviet Psychiatry and Psychology	3
2. Development of Soviet Military Psychiatry	33
3. Soviet Combat Psychiatry in World War II	49
4. Modern Soviet Military Psychiatric Theory	73
5. Preventing Battle Stress	93
6. Soviet Battlefield Psychiatry	121
7. Future Directions of Soviet Military Psychiatry	151
Notes	155
Bibliographic Essay	161
Index	165

Tables

1. Perception of Ideology as an Important Factor in Motivation — 102
2. Important Factors in Fighting Spirit — 103
3. Perceived Quality of Soviet Military Training — 107
4. Perceptions Rating Combat Ability of Soviet Units — 108
5. Drugs Used by Soviet Military Psychiatrists in Treatment of Neurosis and Psychosis — 141
6. Symptom Indicators Used by Soviet Military Psychiatrists to Diagnose Battle Neurosis and Psychosis — 144
7. Common Terms Used in Western Military Psychiatry That Are Not Used by Soviet Military Psychiatrists — 144

Preface

Until very recently, most Western attempts to analyze the Soviet military tended to focus on material or "hard" indicators of military force. Between 1960 and 1980, any number of books and articles were published on the fighting power of the Soviet military using the traditional "intelligence indicators" of military capability, namely, numbers of tanks, artillery pieces, deployment positions, resupply, tactics, and so on. What was missing in almost all of these works was any treatment of what has come to be called the "human dimension of war," those aspects of fighting ability that relate to the ability of the Soviet soldier to stand and fight and to perform his task as well as or better than his Western counterpart.

About five years ago, published works for the first time began to assert that in order to understand the capability of the Soviet military it was extremely important to explore the human factors—morale, cohesion, discipline, fighting spirit, among other things—that are now so crucial in assessing an army's ability to fight. I was fortunate in being able to contribute to this shift in emphasis by publishing *The New Red Legions* (1981, 2 vols.), the first work based on actual interviews with former Russian soldiers. That effort prompted some Western intelligence agencies as well as scholarly establishments to undertake their own larger efforts to systematically interview Soviet emigré populations resident in Western countries with a view toward gaining insights into the mind of the Soviet soldier. Two years later, in 1983, I published *The Antagonists: A Comparative Combat Assessment of the Soviet and American Soldier*, which, for the first time, compared the soldiers of the two primary antagonists along a number of human dimensions of fighting spirit. Shortly thereafter I published *The Mind of the Soviet Fighting Man* which offered the first book comparing a range of human factors as they affected the military performance of Soviet soldiers, sailors, and airmen. These works solidly established the human factor in war as a primary concern of any future analysis of fighting armies.

Although human factor elements are now almost commonplace in studies of the Soviet military, one more element remains to be examined: the functional limits of human endurance under fire. Surprisingly, there is no complete work on the Soviet military's approach to the problem of battleshock as a factor in the equation of military effectiveness. The present work seeks to develop the first comprehensive study of Soviet theory and practice with regard to this subject.

This study has more than academic value. An army's ability both to prevent and deal with psychiatric casualties has had a major role in military effectiveness at least since World War I. In World War II, for example, the American Army lost enough manpower through psychiatric casualties to fill fifty combat divisions, whereas manpower losses for psychiatric reasons amounted to 15 percent of its casualties in Korea and 12 percent in Vietnam. More recently, the Israeli Army lost almost twice the number of soldiers to battleshock in the Lebanese war than were killed by hostile fire. With the advent of nuclear weapons, to say nothing of the increased killing power of conventional weaponry, the ability of an army to prevent and deal with psychiatric casualties will likely be a major element in its ability to achieve victory in even the most conventional of future wars.

Soviet literature offers little help to anyone wishing to study the problem of battleshock in the Soviet Army. Only a handful of published articles on the subject have appeared in Soviet journals, and what little information there is, especially in the overviews offered by the Soviet military every ten years, tends to be incomplete, inaccurate and often, deliberately misleading. Whenever the Soviets approach the subject in print, they paint the Soviet soldier as almost immune to the problem of stress. Equally troubling is the fact that Soviet accounts of the development of psychiatry and psychology in Soviet history are being systematically rewritten for political reasons. Finally, the regime insists that all accounts of psychiatry and psychology square readily with Marxist-Leninist dogma so that even academic debates about the subject within the disciplines themselves are confusing and often so stilted that it becomes impossible to sort out fact from political fancy. Accordingly, the sparse Soviet literature on battleshock is of little help.

The obvious solution is to find psychiatrists and psychologists resident in the West who have had direct first-hand experience with Soviet theory and practice as regards psychiatric casualties. Fortunately, a large Soviet emigré population is readily available. Many of these former Soviet psychiatrists and psychologists are still practicing their disciplines in the West and, as such, are in an excellent position to contrast Western and Soviet theories and practices. Having established extensive contacts with this population as a result of my earlier studies over the last seven years, I found it comparatively simple to locate and interview individuals who had the information I sought.

This book is based on information obtained from interviews with forty-four respondents who have had extensive first-hand experience with the Soviet system of military psychiatry and psychology. The respondents include psychiatrists, psychologists, battle surgeons, public health officials, feldshers (physician's assistants), and medics. Many of these respondents had medical roles in the Soviet Army during World War II, and some occupied comparatively high positions in the Soviet military and civilian medical establishments after the war. Some were very well-published medical practitioners and academics before emigrating to the West, and a few even held academic chairs and official positions in the military medical establishment. The interviews were conducted over a two-year period in the United States, Israel, Canada, and Italy. Finally, a number of the higher ranking respondents consented to read the finished product and to assess it for accuracy and completeness.

Thus, what *Soviet Military Psychiatry: The Theory and Practice of Coping with Battle Stress* offers is the first comprehensive treatment ever published in the West of the Soviet military's approach to the problem of psychiatric casualties. It is my hope that Western military psychiatrists will use this work as a source of information against which to assess their own theories and practices as regards their armies. Moreover, by delineating the seriousness with which the Soviets address the problem, the work may stimulate Western military strategists to pay more attention to stress and breakdown in the development of their own equations of military effectiveness. One thing is certain: psychiatric casualties are inevitable in war, and, as weapons become more destructive, keeping the rates of mental debilitation and degradation down will become critical to the military's ability to fight well. Any military force that ignores this fact is likely to pay a high price.

Acknowledgments

A number of people helped to make this work possible by rendering aid and comfort to the author. Among these is Dr. David Marlowe, chairman of the Department of Military Psychiatry at the Walter Reed Army Institute of Research in Washington, D.C., who saw merit in the work when it was still only an idea. He arranged for my appointment as a Fellow at the institute which allowed me the leisure and resources to complete the research. I am also indebted to Colonel Mike Camp, U.S. Army Medical Corps and Lieutenant Colonel Larry Ingraham, both of the institute, who encouraged me and guided my research by providing answers to innumerable questions about the discipline of combat psychiatry as practiced in the U.S. military.

I am also grateful for the help provided by the professional staff of the Walter Reed Army Institute of Research. In particular, much is owed Colonel Frank Jones, Captain Sam Turner, Major Terry Fullerton, Lieutenant Colonel Bob Schneider, Lieutenant Colonel Paul Furakawa, Colonel Greg Belenky, Professor Joel Teiltelbaum, and Dr. Karen Carney, all of whom read and reviewed the manuscript in detail and who spent three days with me in seminar to examine and critique the work. Also helpful was Dr. Walter Reich of the National Institute of Mental Health and Lloyd Roberts, chief of the Health Sciences Branch of the Foreign Science and Technology Center. I am confident that the comments and critiques offered by these colleagues have made the manuscript a much better book than it otherwise would have been.

Dr. Reuven Gal, chief psychologist for the Israeli Defense Force, and my long-time friend, is owed far too many debts for favors and suggestions to recount here. Thanks is due the U.S. Army Medical Intelligence Center at Fort Dietrick, Maryland, in the person of the overburdened Captain Dick Bloom who took time out from his pressing duties to help me in my research. There is also Bob La Freniere, chief of the Soviet Threat Branch at the Army Intelligence School at Fort Devens who, for two summers, arranged for a comfortable place in which I could conduct my research.

I am also indebted to Paul Corscadden, director of the Center for the Study of Intelligence at the Central Intelligence Agency, for his support and that of my friend and colleague, Professor Larry Black of the Soviet and East European Studies Center at Carleton University in Ottawa who helped track down some of my respondents. Cari Colangelo, my assistant, and Terry Boisenault, my secretary, know well the debt I owe them. Finally, my thanks to St. Anselm College in Manchester, New Hampshire, for providing such a stimulating atmosphere in which to teach and write for the last twelve years. To them, I am especially grateful.

SOVIET
MILITARY
PSYCHIATRY

1
Origins of Soviet Psychiatry and Psychology

This chapter traces the history and development of Soviet psychiatry and psychology as independent disciplines and describes their impact on Soviet military psychiatry up to World War II. It may seem odd to the Western mind to treat Soviet psychiatry and psychology as separate disciplines. Within the United States, both have developed more or less simultaneously, with each complementing the other and each generally welcoming the contributions of the other to its own field. In the Soviet view, American psychology and psychiatry have the same etiological and diagnostic roots which, until recently, have been basically drawn from the theories of Freud as developed by a host of disciples and critics over a period of many years. In the Soviet Union, and in Russia before that, exactly the opposite has been true. Soviet psychiatry and psychology have no common origin or history, did not develop simultaneously, utilize quite different etiological and diagnostic categories, and have been at odds with each other. More importantly, to this day, they remain generally antagonistic to one another.

Whereas in the United States psychology has a long history, in the Soviet Union it remains in the embryonic stages of development. It is at least thirty years behind developments in the United States and faces an uncertain future. In order to understand these conditions and how they affect the development of Soviet military psychiatry and psychology, one must first understand the historical development of each discipline.

For the last hundred years psychiatry in the Soviet Union has been heavily influenced by Germanic schools of thought which teach that the physical operations of the brain as a mechanism underlie the development of mental illness. The Soviets rely on a strict definition of symptoms and the development of precise taxonomies to be used in diagnosis. The goal is to specify the exact biologically determined causes, mechanisms, and manifestations of pyschiatric illness. This basic orientation is called nosological biological psychiatry, and it owes much of its foundation and development to the famous German psychiatrist Emil Kraepelin (1856–1926); its premises spread rapidly to his students and followers in Russia. It was modified and extended, especially in the field of neurosis, by the neurophysiological approach based on the reflexological theories of Ivan Pavlov and Vladimir Bekhterev.

From before the turn of the century until the Soviet Revolution of 1917, most of the top psychiatric practitioners and most of the teaching establishment in Russia were not Russians at all but ethnic Germans. These German professors educated a whole generation of students to their point of view that human emotions and behaviors are rooted in the physiological operations of the brain. These students of the early nineteenth-century transmitted the organic view of behavioral and emotional operations to a second generation of students of psychiatry and psychology. In this regard, one can point to Bekhterev, a great influence on modern Russian psychiatry and founder of the Leningrad School, who was himself educated by German professors. He went on to become, next to Pavlov, probably the most influential figure in Soviet-Russian psychiatry. Another influential Russian psychiatrist, Vladimir Miasishchev, whose career spanned the entire formative period of development of Soviet psychiatry, was also educated by German professors. He received his Ph.D. in the early 1920s, survived the purges and the war, and was responsible for much of the development of Soviet psychiatry until 1948. Still another Russian psychiatrist strongly influenced by the Germanic tradition of psychiatry was Sergei Korsakoff, founder of the Moscow School. His extension of the nosological biological approach to psychiatry is widely known in the West through his description of Korsakoff's psychosis in patients suffering from alcoholic neuropathy. Korsakoff's approach, and that of others of the nosological school, has survived mostly intact in the Soviet Union today and has strongly influenced the development of Soviet psychiatry. The biological orientation of Soviet psychiatry remains the major intellectual pillar on which all of Soviet psychiatry and psychology is based.

The predominance of the Germanic school is reflected in an interesting anecdote. From the early days at the turn of the century until well into the 1900s, the courses taught by German psychiatrists in Russian universities were taught in German or French and not in Russian! As a consequence, the Russian students developed a nickname for their German professors; they called them "nemets," a term that translates as "the mute ones" or, more loosely, those who cannot speak Russian.

The medical somatic approach won the battle between the psychological and biological directions in the study of mental illness which raged in the later 1800s and early 1900s. Accordingly, Russian and Soviet psychiatry considers itself to be a branch of medicine that uses the nosological and biological approach to diagnose and treat disease, including mental illness. Soviet psychiatry is oriented primarily toward the search for the biological causes and mechanisms of psychiatric disease. Psychology is viewed as subservient and a second-rate discipline because its main principles are "brainless," that is, they have no foundation in the physiological operations of the brain. As such, Soviet psychiatrists do not believe that psychology can contribute very much to the scientific and biological foundations of clinical psychiatry. This negative attitude toward psychology was expressed by the famous Russian physiologist, Ivan Pavlov. Pavlov prohibited the use of psychological terms in his laboratory, insisting that they did not reflect any genuine, scientifically provable mechanisms of brain functioning. Today, Soviet psychiatrists believe strongly that American psychiatry's tendency to use the psychoanalytic approach to study psychiatric illness has retarded the development of biological psychiatry in the United States.

Soviet psychiatrists insist that psychology has little in common with psychiatry, especially in dealing with the problems of "big psychiatry," which deals with "genuine" psychiatric disease such as psychosis. Other mental problems, which the Soviets place under "small psychiatry," deal with the diagnosis and treatment of neurosis. Patients with neurosis are not usually treated by a psychiatrist but by neurologists or, in extreme cases, psychoneurologists. The Soviets define the psychiatrist as a medical doctor involved in the diagnosis and treatment of brain disease, especially psychosis.

The system of psychiatric help, hospitals, and outpatient clinics in the Soviet Union operates in such a manner that patients suffering from neurosis would not normally be accepted into the system for treatment except in extreme cases where borderline psychosis might be evident. Although Soviet psychiatrists and neurologists sometimes recognize the role of purely psychological factors in the development of neurosis, as physicians, they tend to focus on the physiological sequelae of such factors, such as the exhaustion or functional disorders of the nervous system. In this way, Soviet clinical psychiatrists try to isolate the "genuine" cases of nervous disease from the flood of patients manifesting neurosis which could easily swamp the medical care system. Although this approach may be economic and particularly effective when used in the field of military psychiatry, it may well leave millions of ordinary citizens with psychological and emotional problems outside the scope of treatment.

It is important to understand that, although Marxism under the Soviets has made its own contributions to Soviet psychiatry, the main thrust of both psychiatry and psychology, namely, the organic and material basis of emotions and behavior, is not an invention of Communist materialism but is a continuation of the main intellectual thrust of Russian psychiatry as introduced by the Germanic school of biological psychiatry at the turn of the century. The Communists imposed on this already extant organic view of psychiatry even more stringent materialist criteria for research and treatment. As a result, the development of psychiatry in the Soviet Union vis-à-vis the West was greatly hampered.

The revolutionary changes, wars, famines, and general social upheavals that affected all of Russia from 1917 to 1945 also profoundly affected Soviet psychiatry and psychology. Psychiatry as a discipline was allowed to develop under the new regime after 1917 because its organic assumptions could be squared with Marxist-Leninist dialectical materialism. Psychology, on the other hand, was almost extinguished as a discipline largely because its focus was on social and "nonrational" explanations of emotions and behavior and clashed openly with the premises of "rationalist" Marxist materialism. Under Stalin, psychology, together with its methodologies, especially testing, was openly denounced and condemned on the grounds that it dealt only with innate intelligence and inherited abilities. Testing and psychological findings tended to contradict Stalinist notions of working-class superiority by demonstrating that bourgeois children, those of higher social class and education, tended to do better on ability tests. Stalin, fearing that these findings would at some point cause major problems of social control, simply outlawed psychological testing. In 1936, a Party Central Committee resolution condemned psychological testing as unscientific and detrimental to the interests of the state. Worse, it sent a clear signal to the members of the discipline that the Party regarded them as enemies to be treated accordingly. As a consequence, since that time psychology in the Soviet Union has been regarded as being in basic conflict with the major Marxist doctrines of material reality. As noted earlier, it will take some thirty years before psychology as an independent discipline can even begin to reemerge as a legitimate area of study in the Soviet Union.

Whereas psychology as a discipline within the Soviet state was almost totally destroyed, psychiatry thrived. Despite Stalinist suppression in almost all other areas of intellectual endeavor, psychiatric practice continued to develop along traditionally organic lines. But the fear of suppression and imprisonment which was characteristic of the entire Soviet society during Stalin's time forced Soviet psychiatry further along in the clinical direction it was already taking. Psychiatrists understood that as long as they kept to clinical applications, that is, practical psychiatry, and stayed away from the larger psychosocial issues, especially those issues addressing the nature of the individual and the emotions, then they were relatively safe. They also understood that the basically Freudian psychoanalytic approaches that were being developed in the United States ran directly contrary to Marxist materialism which underpinned the Soviet state. Any psychiatrist who wandered into this swamp of theoretical and psychosocial questions would, sooner or later, find himself or herself in difficulty and be arrested and imprisoned.

Men such as Ivan Pavlov and Vladimir Bekhterev were taken to heart by the Soviet rulers and laid a scientific and research foundation for Marxist-Leninist applications of theoretical psychiatry, although that was by no means their intent. Today, Bekhterev's work is seen as equal in importance to that of Pavlov and, among clinical psychiatrists, even more so. In the early days, however, the ideas of both Pavlov and Bekhterev were challenged for supremacy in the discipline by others. In the early 1930s, a group called the Red Professors tried to make the main principles of Marxism-Leninism the basis for practical psychiatry. This approach emphasized the role of sociological and economic factors in the development of psychiatric illness. Before long, however, the political authorities realized that with such an approach psychiatric illness would be defined as being caused by the regime's failure to produce the social and economic changes promised by Marxism. By the mid–1930s, a number of the Red Professors were removed from their positions and imprisoned. An interesting aspect of the Red Professor movement was that the works of both Pavlov and Bekhterev were denounced as "vulgar materialism" and removed from medical school libraries. In the mid–1940s, a group of radical Pavlovians offered an extreme version of Pavlov's work as yet another basis for practical psychiatry. But this challenge ended abruptly with the death of Stalin. The more traditional Russian schools of psychiatric thought counterattacked by pointing out that there was little evidence that physiological changes in the brain occurred as a result of conditioned response.

The clinical emphasis of Soviet psychiatry to the neglect of psychoanalytic theory often led to stilted dialogues on how to solve problems. There was a further tendency to begin academic papers and research reports with a bow toward Marxist dogma, a gesture that was intended to demonstrate the consistency of the findings with Marxist assumptions. Once such obeisances had been paid, serious discussions about the clinical applications of the discipline took place. At the same time, terminology began to be used more as a mechanism for squaring practice with Marxist theory than as a way of describing reality. For example, one director of the Bekhterev Institute for thirty years was a true advocate of interpersonal psychiatry as expounded by H.S. Sullivan. Understanding that it would be risky to call his approach psychoanalytic, he simply invented another term for it, psychogenetic analysis. He was able to continue his research for many years without incurring the anger of the regime.

The stress on clinical applications as a consequence of both the pressures of the state and the physiological origins of Soviet-Russian psychiatry, together with the need for practicing psychiatrists to survive, meant that, for almost thirty years, the Soviet psychiatric establishment failed to develop any major new theoretical psychoanalytic approaches to the problems of psychiatric treatment. Instead, it tended to reaffirm the basic organic orientation which rested at the roots of their discipline and to continue its pragmatic clinical approach. As a result, Soviet psychiatry to the present day suffers from a lack of innovative psychoanalytic approaches and models for understanding and dealing with behavioral and emotional problems. In addition, the psychiatric establishment is characterized by a lack of debate on developing new approaches to dealing with human behavior and emotions. On the other hand, Soviet clinical psychiatrists are among the best medically trained and most clinically proficient in the world.

While the Soviet state was suppressing psychology, it openly stimulated the growth of psychiatry, although enforcing a strict direction on it. One way in which the state stimulated the development of psychiatry was to support the research of Pavlov and his experiments with animals dealing with developing conditioned responses. In the late 1940s, the Marxist rulers openly embraced the Pavlovian view of the individual as a product of conditioned responses learned from his or her environment stored and controlled in a rational manner within, what Pavlov called, the second signal system. The focus of psychiatric development and support by the state was along traditional lines of Russian psychiatry buttressed by Pavlov's findings and the layering on of Marxist-Leninist principles addressing the rational nature of materialist man. The state found Pavlov's ideas acceptable for obvious reasons:

It should be recalled that Pavlov's views pointing to a physiological rather than a psychological basis of disorders are particularly acceptable to Marxian materialism because they stress the physiological and rational which fits the Marxian notion of man responsible for his behavior. Freud, on the other hand, emphasized the psychological and irrational. Soviet psychiatry thus endeavors to localize events in the brain, not in the mind. It is frequently held that behind every human action there is a definite physiological occurrence affecting the state of excitation or inhibition in the brain.[1]

Although the organic basis of Russian psychiatry was formed well before the Russian Revolution (Pavlov had received the Nobel Prize for his initial research in 1904), it received added emphasis and direction under the Soviet regime, particularly during the Stalinist era which aided the development of psychiatry by destroying any alternative approaches to the discipline.

Soviet psychiatry maintains its biological and organic orientation, emphasizing that the basic cause of most mental illness, especially psychosis, is organic and that, in time, research data will prove this conclusively. Environmental stress is seen as the primary factor triggering mental aberration in neurosis. Mental illness is, therefore, a question of the disruption of the organic relationships of the physiology rather than the psychology of the mind. There is little question of attributing behavior to irrational or subconscious causes which is so characteristic of Western psychiatry.

Some sense of the importance of biological explanations of mental illness in Soviet psychiatry can be gained from the fact that the term "emotional problem" has no direct equivalent in the Soviet language. Emotional problems are regarded not as entities in themselves, but as symptoms or disorders stemming from physiological causes. Accordingly, when Soviet psychiatrists speak of emotional problems, they usually use the more specific term "nervous disease," which clearly denotes some organic reason for the patient's behavior. In the Soviet psychiatric lexicon, there is no term for assigning emotional problems as the basis for neurosis as is so commonly the case in the West.[2] Soviet biological psychiatry simply does not attribute disruptions of human behavior to nonphysiological problems rooted in the human psyche, which, in any case, cannot be proved to exist because it has no organic properties.

Much of what is done by Soviet psychiatrists is also done by neurologists. In the United States, psychiatrists must first be doctors of medicine. Once they graduate from medical school, complete their tour in psychiatry, and begin to practice, the organic and biological aspects of the practice of psychiatry tend to be subordinated. Most biological psychiatry in the United States, for example, is confined to teaching faculties and research institutions. Until recently, psychiatrists in private practice usually did not emphasize tracing behavioral problems to biological disturbances in the brain. Despite their substantial medical education, until recently

American psychiatrists generally adopted psychoanalytic approaches to behavioral problems and utilized various psychotherapeutic techniques or controlled symptoms rather than look for organic causes of behavioral disruptions.

In the Soviet Union, exactly the reverse is true. Soviet psychiatrists have a strong education in the biological operations of the brain, and it is here that they focus to explain aberrational behavior. Consequently, much of psychiatry in the Soviet Union is really practiced by neurologists. Indeed, the distinction between the two medical specialties is only marginally drawn in a pragmatic sense. This is especially true in the Soviet military. Moreover, Soviet medical education seems particularly designed to produce internists and neurologists. Given the close connection between psychiatrists and neurologists in terms of their basic orientation to the causes of behavioral problems, the emphasis on producing neurologists seems designed to produce a medical doctor who is equally at home in the practice of psychiatry, at least in the clinical setting. The tour in psychiatry to which medical doctors are exposed has a strong biological and physiological orientation in linking behavior to the brain, with almost no time spent on various "bourgeois" theories that link behavior to nonbiological causes. This proved to be of great benefit during World War II when many psychiatrists in the military establishment were neurologists or had a strong neurological background and could adequately diagnose mental problems by pointing to their physiological causes. The other side of this coin, of course, is that Soviet psychiatry has been very slow in developing other aspects of psychiatric practice, namely, psychiatric social workers and counselors. Instead, the focus has remained on biological causes for behavioral disruptions. In examining the clinical psychiatric system as it operates today, it is clear that only a handful of specially educated psychiatric social workers and counselors are available to deal with outpatient problems. When they are found, they are almost always nurses equipped with only primary medical training. Such individuals are likely to have little place in clinical settings.

The growth in psychiatry and neurology in the Soviet Union has been substantial and rapid. In 1960 there were approximately 4,500 psychiatrists and neurologists in Russia. By 1974, that number had grown to 16,000, by 1979 to 19,000, and today probably exceeds

30,000 practicing neurologists and psychiatrists, all of whom are employed by the state. Most psychiatrists apply their skills within research establishments or outpatient mental health hospitals and clinics, and it must be added that the Soviet mental health establishment is indeed quite large. The number of Soviet psychiatrists compared to psychologists (there were fewer than 1,800 in 1974), along with the fact that the regime is still very suspicious of psychology, has guaranteed the Soviet psychiatric establishment a predominant place in the medical-biological and neurological sciences. With this position of power, the psychiatric establishment has been able to direct and even retard the development of Soviet psychology since World War II. As will become clear later, the power of the psychiatric/neurological establishment over the direction and future growth of Soviet psychology as an independent discipline is very great indeed.

SOVIET PSYCHOLOGY

Between 1900 and 1917 and, again in the 1920s, Soviet psychology was in much the same stage of development as psychology in the West. The emphasis was essentially on Freudian emotional, social, and behavioral approaches to human behavior. From the beginning, Soviet psychology did not have strong support among the academic or medical communities largely because its premises flew in the face of traditional Russian doctrine, derived from the German school, that behavior is explainable by changes in the physiology of the brain. (Thus, the charge that psychology is "brainless.") Nonetheless, it seems fair to assert that the number of psychologists in Russia prior to the Revolution was increasing at about the same rate as in the West and that the discipline was taking pretty much the same directions.

With the Soviet Revolution and the disruptions that followed, including the civil war, the war against Poland, and the great famine, Soviet psychology was never quite accepted as a legitimate approach to the problems of human behavior by the rest of the medical establishment. It continued on its own way retarded, perhaps, no more or less in its development than other disciplines. Indeed, the Soviet state had not secured its power sufficiently to impose its ideology on the discipline. This would not happen until

Origins of Soviet Psychiatry and Psychology

1925 with Stalin's collectivization and consolidation of power. In the early 1920s, however, it was already becoming clear that the regime regarded the development of psychology as a potential danger to the state and to the integrity of Marxist philosophy.

The reasons for this are not very difficult to understand. Most psychological approaches at that time emphasized the emotional and subconscious causes of human behavior rather than the objective social or organic causes. It became clear to the regime that such a psychology would ultimately endanger the Marxist view of predictable, rational, conscious, socially dependent human behavior and the historical development of man which would represent a challenge if allowed to survive. By the late 1920s, Stalin had become convinced that psychology was indeed a dangerous discipline, especially psychological testing. The psychological testing mechanisms used in the USSR at that time seem to have been equivalent to those being used in the West. In general, their application was producing the same findings as in the West, namely that factors associated with family environment and training were crucial to later life development and that, on balance, children from bourgeois backgrounds generally performed better than children from working-class backgrounds. Stalin also understood that, in a totalitarian state, he could not allow the existence of any ideology or social doctrine that proposed a competing view of the nature and development of humankind. In 1931, he severely criticized psychological testing, an action that sent a trauma through the discipline; by 1936, the Party formally condemned psychological testing.[3]

Inevitably, the few psychologists in the Soviet Union, and there probably weren't more than a thousand at the time, represented a tempting target for the Stalin purges once the mechanism of repression was set into motion. A substantial number of Soviet psychologists were killed, imprisoned, or forced to recant during the Stalinist Terror. The development of Soviet psychology not only came to a complete halt, but also almost ceased permanently.

When psychology's losses during the Stalinist Terror are added to those it suffered during World War II, it becomes clear that the number of psychologists who survived until 1945 was quite small indeed. Because psychology had been officially discredited, the discipline could not regenerate itself. It had no legitimate place within the academic or medical communities from which it could produce new members. By 1945, the development of psychology as an independent discipline in the Soviet Union was almost dead. Some interest in psychology did survive in the Moscow Institute of Psychology of the USSR Academy of Pedagogical Sciences and in the Institute of Psychology of the Georgian Academy of Sciences, but for the most part, the influence of these institutions declined. The study of psychology as a coherent discipline was kept alive by a handful of psychologists (no more than five) still resident at Leningrad University who had been trained in the old school and who had survived the purges and the war. Among those who managed to survive were Boris Ananyev, chairman of the Department of Psychology at Leningrad in 1948, and later chairman of the Faculty of Psychology at Leningrad University. Another was Vladimir Miasishchev, also at Leningrad University, who had once held a prestigious position at the Bekhterev Institute. Augusta Yarmolenka, a woman whose prewar research in the discipline was widely recognized in the West, also survived and ended up at Leningrad in 1948 where she remained until her death in the mid–1970s. All of these people had been students of Bekhterev before the Revolution. This handful of psychologists preserved the Leningrad branch of Russian psychology during its darkest days and became the primary sources for the development of a new faculty and, eventually, a new discipline in the Soviet Union which finally began to emerge in the 1960s. The group of survivors in Moscow included such luminaries as Alexei Leontiev, A. R. Luria, Boris Teplov, and Bluma Zeigarnik, some of whom, like Luria, reached great heights in the discipline.

Psychology had fallen so low by the end of the war that it even lacked an independent existence. As a clinical and theoretical body of knowledge it had been placed under the philosophical studies program at Leningrad and had almost ceased to exist at any other university. In 1952, Leningrad University graduated its first "majors" in the area of psychology, but under the aegis of the Department of Philosophy. At this time the discipline had no independent faculties or facilities which it could call its own.

As noted above, psychology did not begin to reemerge until the 1960s, when the regime unofficially rehabilitated it. Indeed, the first class of genuine psychologists from any Soviet university was graduated from Leningrad in 1964. This first class graduated only five students! Today only six universities in the Soviet Union offer a genuine degree in psychology; these universities are Moscow University, Leningrad, Tiblisi, Baku, Kiev, and Kalinin. (The University of Tartu in Estonia and the University of Vilnius in Lithuania also offer a degree in psychology.) Since 1968, only about 300 psychology majors each year have been graduated from these universities, and, as of this writing, there are probably no more than 3,000 psychologists in all of the USSR. In 1970, the Soviet Psychological Society listed only 1,800 members, which clearly indicates that psychology as an independent discipline is of comparatively recent vintage.[4]

What factors brought about the "resurrection" of psychology in the 1960s, and who was responsible for it? Interestingly, the stimulus for its resurrection came partly from the military. In 1967, the Soviet military approached Boris Lomov, a student of the surviving psychologists at Leningrad, with the offer of a large grant. The grant was funneled through a number of false institutions in order to cover its military origins. In the Soviet Union these grants are known as "mailbox grants" because the recipient never quite knows the ultimate source of the funding. Lomov was asked to explore the possibility of establishing an institute that would make use of psychology to address a wide range of problems in Soviet life.

In 1967, a number of high-ranking luminaries in the fields of Soviet psychiatry, neurology, and neurophysiology held a meeting at the University of Leningrad, along with the few survivors left in the field of psychology. At that meeting, Lomov suggested the creation of an institute that would explore the possible uses of psychology in tackling a number of problems facing Soviet society. The reception was less than hospitable. A. R. Luria openly opposed the plan. As events turned out, the institute would not be established until 1972 and, even then, only at the strong urging of the military. The idea was tabled in 1967 essentially because of academic politics. Although Lomov had been given the grant, he had also been advised that he would not be the director of the institute because of his lack of seniority in the academic establishment. Thus Lomov, with a reputation in both academic and Party circles as an excellent bureaucratic infighter, began to lay the foundations for the institute between 1967 and 1972, but did not formally establish the organization until he attained sufficient seniority to become director, which he finally did in 1972.

Another indication of the Soviet military's interest in fostering the development of psychology also surfaced in 1967. Then, for the first time, the Soviet military required that a course in psychology be taught in all its military schools, which immediately confronted it with a lack of instructors. The military may simply have been creating a market for the employment of future psychologists. With jobs guaranteed, it could then argue that steps had to be taken to provide the personnel to hold them. The promise of good employment could be used to entice students into the area. At the same time, the regime itself clearly sent a signal that it was ready to countenance a controlled reemergence of psychology when it made psychology courses mandatory for political officers studying at the Political Academy. Despite these initial indications of support from both the military and the political regime, an institute for psychological study was not created for another five years.

In 1972, the Medical Commission of the Academy of Medical Sciences established under its auspices a formal institute for psychological study called the Institute of Psychology of the Academy of Sciences. It was located in Moscow, and Boris Lomov became its director. At this time, a second meeting was held, which included most of the major figures in the field of psychiatry, to discuss the directions the institute would take. The list of individuals attending this meeting comprised the most important and powerful members of the Soviet psychiatric establishment. It included Professor Ivgeny Kuzmin who is professor of psychology in the Central Committee of the Soviet Union. His attendance was a clear indication of the regime's interest in resurrecting psychology as a socially useful discipline. Kuzmin was in charge of implementing the project, and it was he who, in 1967, had been ordered by the Central Committee to begin exploring the possibility of such an institute. Other participants included Alexander Luria and Professor Alexei Leontiev. Luria was chairman of the Department of Neuropsychology at Moscow University, and Leontiev was chairman of the Faculty of Psychology at Moscow University. In addition, Alexei Bodalev, the academic secretary of the Academy of Pedagogical Sciences in Moscow, was also present, as was Konstantine Plantanov, head of the Institute of Philosophy of the National Academy of Sciences. In addition, Miasishchev, former director of the Bekhterev Institute, then a semi-retired but well-respected professor, was present as was Victor Schklovsky, the chairman of the Speech Therapy Center of the Moscow Health District.[5] The gathering together of these luminaries under military guard in which special passes were required for admission suggested that the Soviet military was trying to enlist the support of the powerful psychiatric establishment for the new psychological institute.

The meeting was stormy, and a number of famous participants opposed the establishment of a new institute to direct psychological research. Chief among the opponents was A. R. Luria who was originally trained as a psychologist before obtaining a medical degree. He and other members of the psychiatric establishment opposed the institute on the grounds that it would produce a lot of "junk." He may also have been legitimately concerned that such an institution might siphon off scarce resources into an area of study that was, as yet, unclearly defined and devoid of hard scientific method. Luria's argument focused on the performance of similar institutions in the West which almost uniformly are held in low regard in the Soviet Union. Luria's argument was taken quite seriously inasmuch as he had traveled extensively in the West. He made the strong case that the West had been using the same psychological approaches for years and, he felt, had not accomplished very much except to exclude certain classes from social and economic opportunities. Luria was also concerned that the use of psychological testing mechanisms, especially survey research questionnaires, would lead to an "incorrect understanding" of what truly motivated human behavior. Luria wrote an unpublished report listing his objections and filed it as a minority report. He also obtained the signatures of several other psychiatrists at the meeting who also opposed the institute. Whether he was serious in raising academic and professional objections, Luria understood that with the Party and the military behind the idea, the psychiatric establishment would have to keep a firm hold on the development of psychology or psychiatrists themselves would be challenged for preeminence and influence in the field.

Nonetheless, the institute was established with significant military funding, and its stated purpose was to explore psychological methodologies to address problems in Soviet life. In fact, since its founding the institute has not explored extensive applications of psychological methodologies in any areas that could be regarded as controversial. By and large, it has remained very close to the orientation of its director, Lomov, who holds a degree in engineering psychology. Thus, psychology in the Soviet Union has been channeled into engineering and human factors research, much of it, of course, targeted at military equipment design.

Military support for this project may have been the product of a number of factors, one of which was the desire to emulate or at least keep pace with Western developments in psychology. The Soviet military is acutely aware of progress in the West, and, by the 1960s, Western armies had begun exploring the psychology of the soldier in order to improve the soldier's motivation and performance on the battlefield. The Soviet Army found that it had no equivalent program. Accordingly, the military felt that it had to keep pace even if the directions of progress were not very clear.

Equally important, since World War II, the quality of political officers in the military had risen enormously. The political officer is directly responsible for the morale, motivation, and fighting spirit of the Soviet soldier and his unit. Party support for the project may have been given on the premise that political commissars could, through the use of psychological approaches and methodologies, and morale and cohesion studies (which were very much in vogue in the West at that time) increase the morale and fighting spirit of the Soviet soldier.

Another reason for military support of a psychological institute was probably related to the great doctrinal changes in Soviet military thought between 1967 and 1972. Prior to 1967, the Soviet military's view of war was oriented toward massive nuclear exchanges, essentially massive retaliation. Few members of either the military or the political high command believed that it would be possible to conduct large-scale conventional military operations on a nuclear battlefield. With the fall of Nikita Khrushchev in 1964 and the consolidation of Leonid Brezhnev's power, in the years 1967 to 1970 there was a radical change in the military doctrine of the armed forces: there was a turning back to the experience of World War II. The Soviet military began to believe that it was indeed possible to carry out large-scale conventional operations within a nuclear environment to include theater-level operations. The Soviets seem to have come to believe that such conventional operations, once both sides had exhausted their nuclear arsenals, would probably be decisive.

Whatever the reasons, the Soviet military began to examine the problem of how to increase the soldier's ability to withstand the stress and trauma that would be created in a nuclear environment. Thus, the changes in tactics and strategic orientation that occurred between 1967 and 1972 coincided with the Soviet military's support for the creation and funding of an institute of psychology that could be used to develop psychological approaches in, among other areas, that of military motivation. Although the application of psychological techniques to the study of military morale and "steeling the will" of the soldier is still, by Western standards, in its primitive stages, military support for the resurrection of psychology was no doubt based on the premise that psychology could provide some insight into how to produce a better fighting man in the nuclear age.

In 1985, more than twenty years after the official rehabilitation of psychology in the Soviet Union, it is still not a genuinely independent discipline. In most psychiatric hospitals, psychologists are relatively rare. That there are no psychologists practicing at any level within the Soviet Army, despite military support for reestablishing psychology, shows just how quickly the Soviet military has adopted psychologists. Even where psychologists are found in the Soviet public health system, the psychiatrists and neurologists usually run day-to-day operations and control the activities of psychologists. As in the past, psychologists are not generally allowed to research or administer treatment without the supervision of a psychiatrist. When such "radical" techniques as psychotherapy are attempted, as in the few special experimental psychological clinics for neurosis or in the outpatient mental health centers, public law requires that a psychiatrist or neurologist be present or oversee the treatment. At best, psychology is seen as a research discipline that might someday make some contributions in areas not limited to psychiatry. Even today, members of the practicing psychiatric and neurological establishment do not consider psychologists as legitimate colleagues in the field.

This state of affairs has hampered the development of psychotherapeutic techniques because medical psychiatrists have difficulty accepting them as legitimate treatment methods. There are hardly any psychological research laboratories in medical or psychiatric institutions in the Soviet Union in which psychiatrists do not play a dominant role. Indeed, not until 1968 was the position of psychologist "re-created" as an official job description and position on medical staffs. The rehabilitation of psychology in the Soviet Union since 1967 has proceeded very slowly under the firm guidance of the psychiatric and neurological establishments, which have made no secret of their fear of psychology as a potentially disruptive and even dangerous force.

Some indication of the underdeveloped state of Soviet psychology can be gained from noting that Soviet psychologists did not develop an independent scale for measuring neurosis until 1978. Such a scale was developed in the West in the early 1920s. Furthermore, the use of testing instruments, specifically questionnaires and statistical analysis, is still viewed by most psychiatrists and the regime as ill-proven instruments that are dangerously nonspecific in their applications. The few instruments that exist have mostly been developed in the West, most often in the United States, and have been modified to reflect Soviet values and culture. For example, the Soviets often use the MMPI and Wexler Intelligence Scales adjusted for Soviet values in their research. But even when such instruments are used, they are normally applied within the confines of small rather than large-scale research settings. Apparently, the goal is to develop research models of behavior that can then be used to support extrapolations to larger populations. The research focuses on how people behave under certain circumstances rather than on why they behave. There are few large-scale independent empirical research applications. After all, the use of survey questionnaires by the military, for example, has certain democratic implications: it implies that certain types of social behavior are as acceptable as others, an idea which the regime rejects with a vengeance.

The Soviet psychological establishment is so new that, like any new discipline, it has yet to establish the validity of its approaches and testing mechanisms. For instance, it has not yet been able to agree on appropriate statistical approaches or types of models. As a consequence, most psychological research is conducted within narrow research settings and is still very far from being able to propose applications on a broader scale. It has not even been able to establish adequate data bases that can be used to test and compare research findings for divergent psychological applications.

PSYCHIATRY IN SOVIET LIFE

Of the 30,000 psychiatrists in the Soviet Union, approximately 70 percent of them are women.[6] Soviet psychiatrists study at medical schools for six years in a curriculum of general medical studies. They then undergo one year of internship as general medical doctors and two years of advanced residency training in the area of psychiatry. In general, medical schools offer very little training in psychology per se and only a small number of courses in psychological theory. Considerable attention is given to neuroscience, psychophysiology, and behaviorism as developed by Pavlov. The thrust of the training is traditional biological psychiatry. Psychosis is seen as primarily organic in origin. Environmental stress is most often regarded as a cause of neurosis. Neurosis is attributed to faulty environmental stimuli or the misinterpretation of such stimuli by the organically based second signal system of the individual. There is a heavy emphasis on the findings of Pavlov and Bekhterev, and recently on stress theory, with the works of Freud and other psychic-oriented Westerners regarded as both nonscientific and taboo. Such techniques as psychotherapy and psychoanalytical counseling exist, but generally in an underdeveloped state; they are often found in medically limited environments where they are administered by physicians called psychoneurologists. However, they are generally regarded as too experimental and nonscientific to be taken seriously.

Soviet psychiatric training is narrow in terms of its exposure to publications and research results in psychoanalysis and psychology outside the Soviet Union. In Moscow, where the larger psychiatric institutes are located, there is somewhat greater access to Western materials, but this, too, is carefully controlled and almost never integrated into the instructional curriculum except where it is critiqued. Hospitals outside Moscow and Leningrad have almost no access to modern Western theories and research developments. The result is a fairly narrow education in psychiatry, heavily influenced by biological approaches that stress the organic origins of mental illness. Soviet psychiatrists have access to a monthly magazine that publishes abstracts from Western journals, but, again, only those findings dealing with biological psychiatry are usually included. Access to Western journals is somewhat better if the student is fortunate enough to read German or French. But the students who want translations of English materials or journals will find that, although they are available, they are often restricted, especially articles dealing with psychoanalysis. Students often require formal permission from their faculty directors to gain access to Western materials in libraries. With regard to military psychiatry, experienced Western officers point out that Soviet observers are frequently present at military psychiatric conferences, but their presence is rarely marked by the presentation of papers. Every so often Soviet psychiatrists at these conferences will read a "statement," but almost never do they present their own research results. Apparently, they attend primarily to gather information on Western developments. Soviet psychiatrists collect copies of all papers presented, presumably to bring them back to the Soviet Union for further analysis.

But if it is true that Soviet psychiatric training is only marginally aware of psychoanalytic developments in the West, it may also be said that American psychiatric training is ignorant of developments in the Soviet Union. U.S. psychiatrists often complain that Soviet psychiatrists are completely unaware of advances in American psychiatry when, at the same time, the Americans appear to be as ignorant of Soviet advances in the biological approach to mental illness.

Given the biological premises of Soviet psychiatry, understandably the Soviets have few trained social workers. The clinical and organic orientation of psychiatry all but precludes the use of social workers, so that in health clinics most work is done by psychiatrists rather than by social workers. In Soviet psychiatric clinics there is a greater need to discern and treat the organic causes of behavioral aberrations than to treat "emotional problems." Soviet psychiatrists do not attempt to get the patient to "recognize" his or her problem and "come to grips" with it. Rather, their approach is biological in the sense that they attempt to make the patient "learn" a new response to the particular problem from which he or she may be suffering. It is instructive to point out that the Russian word for "training" is the same as for "learning." In the lexicon of Soviet psychiatry, to train an individual to adjust to certain stimuli or to condition him or her to respond to stimuli in a certain way is the clinical equivalent of having the patient learn to live with the problem.

The physiological base of Soviet psychiatry leads its practitioners to emphasize drug therapies or other physiological cures. In a typical analysis, a psychiatric patient is given a complete medical examination prior to treatment. The Soviet psychiatrist, taking advantage of his or her extensive biological training, is likely to perform tests for hormone levels, blood chemistry, electroencephalograms, brain scans, and other tests aimed at uncovering organic disfunctions. Having found the physical basis for a mental problem, the psychiatrist is likely to treat the problem with a physiologically based therapy. Two commonly used therapies are conditioning, using feedback mechanisms (often hypnosis or other orthogenic training) and drug therapies, through which the patient's physiology is directly altered. With regard to drugs, the Soviets have studied medical drug use in the West in great detail, and are appalled at the large number of patients who seem drug dependent. The Soviet view is that drugs, especially in their military applications, are best used as short-term therapy to disrupt aberrant behavioral patterns. As soon as possible the patient is taken off drugs, which are then replaced by natural compounds until drug use can be abandoned altogether. During this time the patient develops new conditioning patterns that finally alter his or her behavior. The Soviets are, therefore, far less likely than the United States to use long-term drug therapy in dealing with psychiatric cases.

Certain elements of Soviet psychiatric practice are remarkably similar to those used in the West. For example, in 1982 at Moscow Clinic #5, operant therapy was used for the first time in the Soviet Union, although this technique has been used in the West for almost sixty years.[7] The treatment of neurosis in such special clinics (there are only a few, perhaps no more than four or five for inpatient treatment of neurosis as of 1985) is highly experimental and includes short-term drug therapy, biofeedback, physical massage, group therapy, sensitivity sessions, counseling, and even therapeutic dance. Although some of these techniques are premised on psychoanalytic assumptions, the search for the organic cause of behavioral aberration continues, and almost always leads to physiological treatment through drug therapy, relearning, or conditioning. The Soviet psychiatrist believes that people are totally malleable to a set of objective social conditions, and the focus on the organic causes of behavioral problems plays down any consideration of psychic and subjective causes. Rather than seeing traumatic neurosis as the subjective interpretation of the event itself, the Soviet psychiatrist would argue that the objective event has an objective impact on the organism, which sets up a physiological disruption, and that the subjective aspects of it are not nearly as important. Therefore, stress-related problems will likely go untreated while the psychiatrist treats only the more overt symptoms.

A final difference between the U.S. and Soviet approach to the success of treatment is that whereas U.S. psychiatry stresses the necessity of building the psychiatrist-patient relationship based on mutual trust and confidentiality, in the Soviet Union, it is very difficult to establish such a relationship in a clinical sense, especially in treating neurosis. Individuals are acutely aware that there is no private psychiatric practice and that whatever passes between a patient and a psychiatrist will become part of a permanent record in the public health system that may at any time be used against the patient. Therefore, the development of any kind of large-scale outpatient psychiatric therapy modeled on Western lines is out of the question.

The Soviet Union has no tradition of individualized psychiatric care; every psychiatrist works for the state public health system. Moreover, patient visits become part of one's psychiatric record, which is kept on file as a public document in the public health clinic. Since 1975, such data has been collected by catchment area and assembled in a centralized computerized file in Moscow where they are used for research purposes. Clearly, a centralized computer file of mental health patients is subject to potential political abuse, and there is every reason to suspect that, in difficult times, such information may be used against a patient.

In addition, being labeled a person with a psychiatric problem carries greater social stigma in the USSR than it does in the United States. A psychiatric record can make life miserable for those who are guilty of any political or social deviation, for it can lead to the placement of such individuals in psychoprisons. In the Soviet Union individuals who, in the West, would be regarded as guilty of simple political opposition, are regarded as truly psychotic and are sent to special psychiatric prisons where they are subject to a number of therapies, such as heavy drug use, electric shock treatment, and isolation, that seem almost punitive rather than curative in purpose.

When an individual ventures into a psychiatric clinic, thus initiating a personal psychiatric record, there can be severe implications for that person's day-to-day life. For example, any Soviet citizen seeking to travel abroad, especially to the West, must obtain a certificate from the local psychiatric dispensary testifying to his or her mental stability. The certificate is required even if there is no history of psychiatric care in order to prove that one does not have such a history! Although there are ways in which psychiatric records can be expunged, usually by bribing a clerk in the clinic, such a record usually follows the individual for a very long time. The application for a driver's license also requires a certificate testifying to one's mental stability, or at least the lack of a psychiatric record. Thus, the certificate of psychiatric stability and its corollary, the certificate of psychiatric history, is an integral part of the Soviet internal control system. The system of centralized psychiatric records gained great momentum after 1970 with the increased number of psychologists and the computerization of medical records on a country-wide basis. There is now a self-generating bureaucracy which collects and maintains these records. Hence, psychiatric care in the Soviet Union cannot be kept confidential. Referrals to psychiatric clinics may come from the individual involved, from other clinics, medical doctors, schools, the work place, or even the police. Any agency of the state can refer a client for psychiatric evaluation.

Soviet society and the regime enforce a view of life that tends to denigrate the use of psychological reasons as a way of avoiding social responsibility. In a typical Russian rather than Soviet way, the regime imposes a perspective that sees life as difficult, requiring a degree of hardship and suffering as normal conditions in a society surrounded by hostile states. The traditional Russian belief that life is hard and that it is the individual's responsibility to adjust to it is as much alive under the commissars as it was under the czars. As a consequence, mental disability is not regarded as a legitimate excuse for failure to perform one's job or family obligations. Rather, Soviet society is likely to perceive an individual with a neurotic problem as one who has willfully made an adjustment in order to avoid responsibility. Either that, or he or she is just faking. Schizophrenia, for example, is defined as a citizen's inability to adjust to the objective realities of society which are themselves historically and objectively determined. Because objective realities are just that, namely, determined by forces quite outside the individual, then the responsibility for adjustment rests with the individual, not with the society itself which in the United States is said to need changing in order to reduce pressures on the individual and thereby prevent psychiatric breakdown. Responsibility for proper behavior is focused upon the individual citizen, not on irrational or subconscious emotional forces or even upon objective social forces themselves.

This perception of focused individual responsibility has led Soviet psychiatry to a much smaller role in the correction of social behavior than other forces. Accordingly, many psychiatrists are employed in the diagnosis and treatment of patients with clearly defined psychosis. A great deal of emphasis is placed on psychiatric research and the proper training of individuals for certain jobs or on conditioning individuals away from certain patterns of behavior or toward others. The Soviets also emphasize pedagogical or educational systems wherein psychiatric evaluations are seen to play a considerable role. As noted above, Soviet psychiatric thought proceeds from the assumption that human beings are infinitely malleable in a Marxist sense, and much of Soviet psychological research is therefore directed at developing ways in which people can be made to conform to the objective social realities that history presents. The Soviet commitment to developing a citizen with a new nature ought not to be dismissed by Western analysts as ideological nonsense. The idea of changing human nature is, to the Western mind, at once the most intriguing and most distasteful thrust of psychiatric practice in the Soviet Union. In the eyes of the regime, the psychiatrist is the servant of the state whose task it is to treat those individuals who deviate from objective social realities or cannot adjust to them. The objective of psychiatric treatment is to get the patient to accept the objective conditions under which he or she is expected to function, and to get on with his or her responsibilities as a citizen. The thought of using psychiatric research to question the applicability of certain mechanisms of social control or any other social institution is totally foreign to psychiatry in the Soviet Union.

THE SOVIET PSYCHIATRIC ESTABLISHMENT

It is possible to piece together, however imperfectly, a picture of the Soviet psychiatric and psychological research establishment. Many Soviet psychiatrists and psychologists work in research rather than in clinical roles, although the number of psychiatrists in clinical roles is very large indeed. The number of psychiatric beds in the USSR exceeds that of the United States by almost two times, and the number of district psychiatric clinics dealing primarily with psychosis exceeds that of the United States by almost four times. The future of Soviet psychiatry in the field will be determined essentially by the directions of research in the major research establishments. A review of the literature and extensive interviews with former Soviet psychiatrists, some of whom worked for these establishments, reveals a number of major research organizations that are worthy of attention: the Department of Psychiatry at the Kirov Military Medical Academy in Leningrad; the Institute of Psychology of the Soviet Academy of Medical Sciences; the USSR Institute for Industrial Design (known by its initials as VNITTE); the Pharmacology Laboratory of the Psycho-Neurological Research Institute located at the Bekhterev Institute; the Institute of Higher Nervous Activity and Neurophysiology located in Moscow. Although there are other institutions that carry out psychological and psychiatric research, these five are the focus of the new research being conducted in the Soviet Union.

The Kirov Military Medical Academy in Leningrad is the preeminent military psychiatric institute in the USSR. It is the chief institution for training military doctors and psychiatrists. However, it does not appear to play a very large role in psychiatric research. Even the psychiatric research undertaken directly by the military seems to be conducted largely at the Institute of Psychology of the Soviet Academy of Sciences. Nonetheless, the Kirov Academy is charged with producing military psychiatrists who would deal with battle casualties. It is also the focus of most other military medical developments in the Soviet Union, although VNITTE performs a considerable amount of new work for the military.

The Kirov Academy, founded in 1802 as a medical surgical academy, is the oldest military medical school in the Soviet Union. It became identified with the military well before the outbreak of

World War I. The chairman of the Department of Psychiatry at Kirov is General Leonid Spivak who replaced General Nicolai Timofeev in 1977. In 1975, Timofeev made the initial overture to the Bekhterev Psychoneurological Institute to obtain instructors to conduct what the Soviets call an "expertise" or symposium in psychological research at the Kirov Academy. However, the military does not have its own psychologists for research purposes, although it does have a small number of psychiatrists. In the mid–1970s, the Bekhterev Institute was approached to have psychologists present papers at the Kirov Academy; this was one of the strong indicators at the time of official military interest in psychology with possible military applications. In addition, a number of psychiatrists were sent to the Bekhterev Institute for medico-psychological training. Although the Kirov Academy is the chief locus of military psychiatric and psychological interest in the Soviet Union, there are still no psychologists on the staff of the Department of Psychiatry. To this day psychology is taught by psychiatrists who have taken a number of additional courses at the Bekhterev Institute. In any case, the Kirov Academy is the highest staff level of the Soviet military medical establishment. Its partial equivalent in the United States is the Department of Military Psychiatry at the Walter Reed Army Institute of Research in Washington, D.C.

A second major psychological research establishment is the Institute of Psychology of the Soviet Academy of Sciences in Moscow. As discussed earlier, this organization was created in 1972 at the direction of the Party, with funding from the military. Its original goal was to explore and coordinate the development of psychological approaches to problems in all areas of Soviet life. Its present task, however, is to coordinate all psychological research efforts in the Soviet Union. Although its director, Lomov, is primarily an engineer, he is also a graduate of Leningrad University, class of 1952, when psychology was still under the aegis of the Department of Philosophy. Lomov has directed the emphasis of the institute toward engineering and other human factors research to include the operation and design of military equipment. The institute itself has a staff of 800 people and is divided into five major departments, none of which deals directly with the problem of military psychology or psychiatry.[8] Apparently, the problem of treatment and prevention of psychiatric breakdown in the Soviet soldier is handled exclusively at the Kirov Academy. Most of the institute's staff are psychiatrists and neurologists, although the number of psychologists is growing. Only a handful are psychologists, and on the basis of interviews with individuals who used to work there, it may be concluded that the few psychologists have little influence and direct no major research projects. This control and distrust of psychologists seems to be characteristic of the entire research establishment and reflects the historical and continued dominance of neurologists and psychiatrists in the field with their physiological orientation toward behavioral problems.

If the Institute of Psychology is concerned primarily with the psychophysiological problems in operating and designing equipment, its natural corollary is the USSR Institute for Industrial Design located in Moscow and directed by Uri Solobyov. This is the largest human engineering research facility in the Soviet Union, employing 500 people in Moscow and another 1,500 in nine branch institutes spread throughout the country.[9] Yet, for all its manpower, the Institute for Industrial Design houses only forty psychologists. Most of the staff are engineers. This institute acts as a clearinghouse for all human engineering research and development. Once again, there is only a marginal emphasis on true psychological applications, and, even here, the emphasis remains on the physiological reactions of individuals to certain specified mechanical operations.

On balance, Soviet human factors research, as it is called in the West, is still way behind similar efforts in the West. According to one intelligence estimate, about 35 percent of this research is targeted at equipment design.[10] This approach poses little risk to either the regime or the psychiatric establishment which has a tendency born of experience to avoid controversial theoretical issues. Sixty-five percent of the research effort is concerned with operator selection and training and here the focus until most recently has been on pilots, astronauts, and submariners.[11] According to former staff members of the institute, little effort is devoted to the problem of human motivation in carrying out mechanical operations, and almost none to the problem of motivating the soldier.

For the Soviets, human psychological engineering is far more concerned with the physical interactions of men and equipment, with only slight emphasis on the psychic or emotional components. When the research does address mental interactions of men and machinery, the focus tends to be on the problem of degradation of performance as a consequence of fatigue or stress. This approach reflects the traditional view of "consciousness as action" residing in the higher nervous system as a result of conditioned response. As such, it avoids the range of problems that are not purely physiologically based and that might bring research efforts into direct conflict with the premises of the regime itself.

Three additional research establishments are worth noting, but little is known about their operations. The first is the Pyschopharmacological Laboratory of the Moscow Institute of Psychiatry of the USSR Department of Health. This organization was founded in the early 1960s and was formerly headed by I. P. Lapin and, more recently, by G. Y. Avrutsky. Avrutsky is among the best known psychopharmacologists in the Soviet Union, whereas Lapin is known for his work in the theory of depression. That this is one of the oldest pharmacological institutes in the country is a clue as to the relatively recent state of pharmacological research in the Soviet Union. Nonetheless, in the last decade, through a combination of their own efforts and their adoption of drug technology developed in the West, the Soviets have moved ahead very rapidly in this area. This institute apparently emphasizes the use of pharmacological agents to prevent and counter stress-related illnesses. Although the military applications are obvious, a review of the extant literature, both in the West and the Soviet Union, reveals little evidence of widespread military application of drug therapies to prevent stress. This subject is addressed in greater detail later; suffice it to say here that what drug-related approaches are discernible in the military appear to be primarily in the research stage and confined to small research applications. As yet, there has been no widespread application of drug programs to prevent battle stress.

One of the more interesting and highly secret institutes dealing with psychiatric and psychological research in the Soviet Union is located within the Institute of Toxicology in a large building directly next to the Bekhterev Institute in Leningrad. The institute originated in the early studies of poison gas and other toxins with military applications done almost fifty years ago in Russia. Since then, it has expanded considerably, and has become the primary institution for the study and development of military pharmacology. Its present focus seems to be on the development and testing of militarily useful chemicals, including studies in psychological drugs designed to alter mental states, general microtoxins, and paralytic gases. The grounds of the institute are guarded, and access is carefully controlled, although from time to time, the Bekhterev Institute has been asked to replicate results by testing them on psychiatric patients. The director of the Institute of Toxicology is Professor A. A. Krilov.

Another major research institute is the Institute of Higher Nervous Activity and Neurophysiology located in Moscow and currently headed by Professor Pavel Simoniov who replaced its first director, Professor Ashraf Asratyan, in the mid-1970s. The existing literature does not reveal its precise activities, but interviews with former employees indicate that it is concerned primarily with animal behavior. Simoniov himself is a specialist in the physiology of emotion. The approach seems to be essentially Pavlovian inasmuch as the Soviets regard higher nervous activity as equal to consciousness. Whatever research has been conducted on the alteration of consciousness as it relates to military applications is highly classified, but may be presumed safely to be on the cutting edge of the field.

SUMMARY

The Soviets continue to be apprehensive about psychology as an independent discipline, for they fear it will eventually bring it into conflict with Marxist doctrine as well as clinical biological psychiatry and neurophysiology. Both disciplines must also exist within the confines of a totalitarian state which vigorously proselytizes and defends an ideological view of humankind which it must maintain at all costs if it is to continue to justify its nature. Consequently, both psychology and psychiatry must function within a social, clinical, and intellectual straitjacket that often limits and prohibits areas of research to those subjects considered safe by the regime.

Psychology's present rate of development is being watched cautiously and directed slowly into noncontroversial areas, most often into industrial and engineering uses. As a discipline, it is still grossly underdeveloped in terms of controlling its own resources, with the first class of genuine psychologists having been graduated from university less than twenty years ago. Psychiatrists still maintain a dominant role in all the psychological research establishments and frequently conduct psychological research themselves. Finally, the psychiatric establishment by no means agrees that psychology should be allowed to be a separate discipline with its own resources and its own operating assumptions. Many of the powerful figures within the psychiatric establishment in the postwar period are still in a position to retard the development of psychology and are apparently quite willing to do so. Psychology has yet to acquire the legitimacy as a valid social science that it enjoys in the West.

For the foreseeable future, say the next two decades, psychology in the Soviet Union will likely remain an underdeveloped research discipline continually meeting resistance from other sectors of the medical and political establishments for a larger, more encompassing applied social and clinical role of its own. Psychiatry, on the other hand, will no doubt continue to prosper because its biological and medical orientation and clinical applications were long ago made congruent with Marxist ideology and the regime's more pragmatic goals. The regime does not regard the practice of psychiatry as a threat to its control, and the members of the psychiatric establishment have already proven themselves able to sustain their research and practice without threatening the basic assumptions of Marxist-Leninism which underpin the totalitarian state. Indeed, given the recent development and use of psychoprisons which, in the view of many Soviet psychiatrists make ultimate sense, psychiatry may have found yet another role to play which will endear it to the regime and thus further secure its future.

2
Development of Soviet Military Psychiatry

Like all things Russian, military psychiatry in its present form has been enormously influenced by the experience of the Russian and Soviet armies on the field of battle. Soviet military history has been marked by the slow learning of past lessons and their gradual adoption in order to develop solutions to modern problems. The Soviets have shown a marked tendency not to depart radically from the lessons of past wars, and, in a number of areas, they are considerably behind modern developments because their focus is on their last battle experience. Although all armies generally tend to plan for the last war, this tendency seems particularly characteristic of the Soviet military. Their clinging to the experiences of the past is evident in their philosophy of equipment design, tactics, strategy, utilization of the soldier, and many other areas. It is no less evident in the field of military psychiatry. Therefore, in order to place modern Soviet military psychiatry in perspective, it is helpful to be aware of the historical development of Russian military psychiatry from the turn of the century through World War II.

1900–1917

The first army to specifically diagnose mental disease as a consequence of the stress of modern warfare and to attempt to do something about it was the Russian Army during the Russo-Japanese War of 1905. Earlier, as with the British in the Boer War and the Americans in the Civil War, soldiers who manifested behavioral problems affecting their ability to fight were identified. But their problems were generally attributed to factors other than the sheer stress of combat. In the American Civil War, for example, many behavioral problems were blamed on something called nostalgia or homesickness, whereas in the Boer War many of the behavioral problems shown by British soldiers were traced to nutritional deficiencies and physical disease. A common practice during these early days was to attribute the mental problems of soldiers to cowardice or lack of character, a practice that endured in some Western armies through World War II. Although the American, French, and British armies in World War I attempted to deal with battle stress as a cause of mental collapse, in practice, it was generally held that fear, anxiety, depression, hysteria, malaise, and other such problems were due essentially to defects in the soldier's character or training.

During the Russo-Japanese War, physicians in the Russian Army diagnosed and treated approximately 2,000 casualties which they directly attributed to the stress of battle and its resulting psychiatric breakdown. But the number of soldiers complaining of psychiatric symptoms was much larger, so large in fact that they overburdened the medical system and were shipped home and turned over to the Russian Red Cross Society for institutionalized care. The number of neuropsychiatric casualties reached such proportions that even the home front resources proved eventually to be insufficient. The Russian experience in 1905 provided the first example of "evacuation syndrome" in modern times. When soldiers began to realize that "insane" soldiers were being evacuated, the number of psychiatric casualties increased dramatically.

The Russians seem to have been the first to place psychiatrists relatively close to the battlefront in order to deal with psychiatric breakdown. Most of these psychiatrists, however, came from civilian mental hospitals and had no training in dealing with military psychiatric problems. Psychiatric dispensaries staffed with psychiatrists and other medical personnel were established near the front lines and had their own transport, usually a specially marked ambulance, to deal with stress casualties as distinct from physical casualties.[1] The dispensary staff often included a neurologist, a feldsher, and three sanitors (medics) under the direction of a psychiatrist. Although most Western armies reached this degree of organizational definition by 1917, the principle of proximity—stationing psychiatric personnel close to the battlefront and treating neuropsychiatric casualties there—was a practical lesson that seems to have been forgotten during the interwar period and did not reemerge in practice until the later days of World War II. It reappeared in full form in Korea and later in Vietnam when it was used by the American Army. After the 1973 war in Israel, the Israeli Army sent experts to the United States to study American doctrine and practice concerning the problem and, between 1974 and 1983, established a doctrine and structure for treating stress casualties closely based on the American model.[2] On balance, however, the Russian Army in 1905 was the first to develop the practice, if not the theoretical underpinning, of a basic premise of military psychiatry: the principle of proximity of treatment. Their performance, however, was marginal because, in fact, little forward treatment of psychiatric casualties was accomplished.

In the Russo-Japanese War, the Russian Army established a central psychiatric hospital behind the lines in the town of Harbin, Manchuria. This hospital recorded between forty-three and ninety admissions a day for neuropsychiatric casualties. Of these, only a few could be rapidly treated and sent back to the front. Those who remained in the hospital did so for about fifteen days where they were subjected to a variety of treatment therapies. If they did not recover, they were then evacuated to Moscow by train, a trip that often took forty days because only a single railroad track ran from Harbin to Moscow.[3] Evacuation was accompanied by a surgeon and a small staff of feldshers, and, by the end of the war, the Russian Medical Corps had established a number of special trains exclusively for the use of psychiatric patients. These trains had special isolation compartments, restraint rooms, and barred windows in order to control the patients.[4]

Although the Russians attempted to treat psychiatric casualties at the front, the rates of successful recovery suggest that the treatment was not very successful. Of the 275 officers admitted to the psychiatric hospital in Harbin during the war, only fifty-four recovered sufficiently to be sent back to the lines, whereas 214 were evacuated to Moscow. Of the 1,072 enlisted soldiers treated in Harbin, only fifty-one recovered and were returned to their units and 983 were evacuated to the rear.[5] Even in 1905 the Russians began to recognize the problem of secondary gain. They discovered quickly that the further a soldier suffering psychiatric symptoms was evacuated from the front, the less likely he was to recover from his symptoms. Secondary gain is due to a number of factors. In the Russian view, it was due to the perception that stress reactions were often functional for the soldier in that they allowed him to escape the horrors of battle. Once the soldier understood that certain symptoms would allow him to be evacuated out of danger, he began to manifest those symptoms. Moreover, as he was moved further and further away from the battle area, his ability and willingness to reverse those symptoms decreased, so that the further to the rear he went the deeper his symptoms became. Secondary gain became a major problem for Western armies in World War I and World War II. By the end of World War I, the experience of most Western armies had confirmed the validity of the Russian experience with secondary gain in 1905.

During the Russo-Japanese War, Russian physicians appear to have made significant advances in linking battle stress with certain types of somatic symptoms. If one analyzes the diagnoses of hundreds of psychiatric cases during the 1905 war, one finds that the Russians were already able to diagnose battle stress casualties by categories that are quite modern. Russian psychiatrists recorded cases of hysterical excitement, confused states, fugue states, hysterical blindness, surdomutism, local paralysis, and neurasthenia.[6] Although they understood that these symptoms were related to battle stress, Russian psychiatrists, drawing on their own German medical education, tended to define the impact of stress in purely physiological terms. Thus, a wide range of battle stress symptoms were attributed to traumatic psychosis of organic origins. In the Russo-Japanese War, 55.6 percent of the battle stress casualties were attributed directly to traumatic damage to the brain or the nervous system.[7]

By the end of the Russo-Japanese War, and certainly by World War I, the Russian Army probably had the most practical clinical experience in dealing with stress casualties insofar as it recognized stress per se as a cause of psychiatric disability. To be sure, by modern Western standards its treatment methods would be regarded as somewhat primitive, but for their time they were comparatively advanced. The Russo-Japanese War also provided physicians in the Russian Army with the first practical opportunity to institutionalize clinical treatment methods for stress casualties deduced directly from the organic and physiological premises of Russian biological psychiatry. Thus, the mold was set for continuing the physiological approach to the treatment of battle stress that would persist until the present in the Soviet Army. By defining psychiatric disorders as a disease resulting from physiological damage, Russian military physicians differed from their Western counterparts who, after 1917, persisted for almost forty years in attributing stress breakdown to cowardice or deformations in the soldier's character. Finally, the Russian experience in the Russo-Japanese War established a significant experiential base for institutionalizing the principle of proximity of treatment as a way of dealing with the greater problem of secondary gain.

WORLD WAR I

The experience of the Russian Army with battle stress in World War I remains obscure. It is simply not possible to reconstruct that history in any great detail from available sources in the West or, indeed, even from those available to Soviet scholars themselves. Apparently, little Russian literature on the subject of battle psychiatry has survived.

The reasons are obvious enough. Most literature related to war emerges only after a war is over. During wartime, communication is limited for reasons of national security and the obvious obstacles to normal academic or intellectual intercourse. Furthermore, the period following World War I in Russia was marked by events so severe and traumatic as to make the collection and publication of information on almost any scientific or medical subject very difficult and, in many cases, impossible. Following the destruction of World War I in which 11 million Russians, military and civilians, died, the entire society was shaken to the core by the Soviet Revolution of 1917. Between 1917 and 1920, the civil war claimed another 4 million lives. Between 1917 and its reconstitution in 1927, the Russian/Soviet Army ceased to exist as a national entity. Finally, many of the psychiatrists and neurologists were drawn from the upper and bourgeois classes of Russia and, as such, were killed during the civil war. Taken together, these events alone would have been enough to ensure that the collection and transfer of information about Russian battle psychiatry would be minimal.

In addition, between 1921 and 1922 Russia suffered through a great and devastating famine. Historians note that this famine was probably the most severe famine in the history of the country. Although the exact figures cannot be substantiated, it is estimated that the number of dead due to starvation during the postwar famine exceeded the total number of dead in both the civil war and World War I![8] If so, this means that upwards of 15 million Russians died from hunger and hunger-related disease in a two-year period. Also contributing to the paucity of psychiatric research and information available in that period was the emigration of more than 2 million people from Russia, many of them members of the intellectual, academic, and medical elite. In 1922, the Soviets embarked on a disastrous war against Poland which cost several hundred thousand dead and wounded. In 1928, Stalin began his infamous collectivization plan in which another 5 to 8 million Russians would eventually lose their lives. In the early 1930s, Stalin instituted the Great Terror, a period of remarkable brutality that eventually claimed 8 million lives. Finally, in 1939 the war against the Finns produced more deaths and further social disruption.

Thus, between 1917 and 1940, the period in which one would have expected that much of the Russian experience with battle psychiatry in World War I would have finally emerged in print, there is no material available on the subject at all. If one searches the international medical journal, *Lancet*, as well as Russian medical journals from 1914 to 1940, not a single article is found from any source dealing with the subject of Soviet or Russian military psychiatry or the treatment of neuropsychiatric casualties in World War I.

None of this means that physicians in the Soviet Army were not thinking about the problems of military psychiatry. In their official histories, which must always be regarded with some distrust especially in the area of psychiatry, the Soviets note that between 1918 and 1920 three books a year were published on the general subjects of psychology and psychiatry. Between 1931 and 1940, their official histories list seven books a year published on the subject.[9] Yet, an examination of these works shows that all were highly theoretical and dealt far more with the problem of trying to square Marxist ideology with the clinical approaches of military psychiatry than with actual techniques of the discipline. By and large, the works centered on the psychology of military teaching.

Between 1921 and 1940, the Kirov Military Medical Academy in Leningrad continued its work in the area of military psychiatry and psychology, focusing on military teaching and training. These problems were important for the Party inasmuch as the Red Army was regarded as a totally new social institution comprised of workers and peasants based on its own unique psychology of Marxist-Leninism. As with psychiatry and psychology in the society as a whole, military psychiatry was affected by the same swings in Party positions that affected the discipline and was marked by a continuing attempt to resolve the tension between bourgeois and Marxist approaches to human nature. In the case of military psychology, the tension initially resolved itself in the death of the discipline when Stalin simply outlawed it.

It should also be mentioned that the political purges took a high toll of the old intellectual elite, including civilian and military doctors, psychologists, and psychiatrists. After Stalin made it clear in 1936 that he regarded psychology as dangerous to the political consciousness of the citizenry, in the words of a Soviet journal, "a sharp reduction in research in military psychology occurred in practice. Only in military aviation psychology were high rates of research maintained."[10] Only as the purges tapered off and World War II was about to begin did the Party realize that it had need for a developed doctrine of military psychiatry and psychology. In January 1941, the People's Commissariat for the Defense of the USSR raised the question of the need to develop a military psychology to "create psychological bases for combat and political training."[11] By then it was too late, and World War II broke out a few months later.

Despite the difficulty in obtaining hard data on Soviet psychiatric practice in World War I, one may gain some insight into how the Russian Army handled the problem by remembering that much of their medical practice during the war strongly paralleled their own experiences in the Russo-Japanese War. In addition, most Russian psychiatric practice was, at base, German psychiatric practice and probably so in the military sphere as well. Many techniques that surfaced in World War II were imitations of techniques used by the German Army in World War I. Accordingly, Russian psychiatric practice in World War I most probably used such basic techniques as electric stimulation of paralyzed limbs, water therapy, rest, and folk medicine derivatives and stimulants.[12] The Germans used all of these techniques in World War I, and the Red Army still used them in World War II. Beyond such general statements, not much can be said about Russian psychiatric practice in World War I. It has taken this writer almost two years of research to piece together even a partial history of the development of Soviet military psychiatry during World War II.

WORLD WAR II

Before we can assess the Soviet Army's ability to handle battle stress casualties in World War II, it is first necessary to establish a baseline against which the data can be analyzed. This task is complicated by the fact that the Soviets have been very secretive about much of their battle performance in the Great Patriotic War and, since 1950, have been engaged in an effort to rewrite much of what happened into their own version of history. There is only one known document that chronicles the activities of the Soviet medical corps in World War II. In 1948, a multi-volume work entitled *The Experiences of Soviet Medicine in the Great Patriotic War* was published. A complete volume was given over to the treatment of psychiatric cases.[13] Unfortunately, the work is not available in the West and, in recent years, has even disappeared from the shelves of Soviet medical libraries. This writer has been fortunate to be able to locate a number of former Soviet military physicians who have read this work, but it has been impossible to gain access to the original document. The material presented in this chapter is therefore based largely on interviews with individuals who served during World War II in the Soviet medical corps.

Western military analysts have not reached a consensus as to exactly how many men the Soviet Union mobilized for military service in World War II. There is further disagreement about the number of dead and wounded which the Soviet Army suffered in that war. T. R. Dupuy in his *Encyclopedia of Military History* states that the Soviets mobilized 25 million men for battle in World War II, and of that number 7.5 million were killed and another 14 million wounded.[14] These numbers suggest that almost everyone who served in the Soviet military during the war was either killed or wounded! A second casualty estimate is offered by Lieutenant Colonel Robert Glantz of the Strategic Studies Institute of the U.S. Army War College, Carlisle Barracks, Pennsylvania. Glantz suggests that Dupuy's figures are too high, and he argues that the Soviets mobilized about 20 million men, of whom 5 million were killed and between 8 million and 9 million were wounded.[15] Whichever estimate one accepts, the fact remains that the number of men mobilized, killed, and wounded in the Soviet military was enormous. Unable to resolve the conflict between the two figures definitively, it seems useful for purposes of this analysis to choose a figure somewhere between the two estimates and to use the figure of 22 million as a baseline for determining the number of Soviet citizens conscripted for military service in World War II. Of this number, almost 20 million were eventually put in uniform.

By contrast, the United States conscripted approximately 20 million men for military service. Of these, 14 million passed the initial physical and psychological screening and were eventually pressed into military service. Of these 14 million soldiers, 260,000 were killed and another 480,000 were wounded. In terms of military psychiatry, it is interesting to note that of the 14 million U.S. soldiers, about 502,000 suffered psychiatric problems of sufficient magnitude to allow them to obtain a release from military service.[16]

During World War II, the United States adopted as its standard for military service the requirement that a conscript be "fit for combat," thereby exempting anyone who could not pass this test. Little or no thought was given to conscripting people who could be used in limited military roles, even though they could not handle the rigors of the battlefield. The Soviets apparently had no formal philosophy or standard of selection save that of the obvious physical impairments that would normally exempt anyone from strenuous exercises as well as combat. Their basic philosophy of recruitment was that every Soviet citizen, including women, had to serve in some capacity. There were no nonmedical exemptions from military service. Nor were any psychological or behavioral models used to screen conscripts as was the case in the West. In practice, there was no definitive philosophy of screening at all. Everyone was expected to serve, and soldiers were assigned where needed and were expected to perform. When they failed to perform, harsh punishments, often death, were imposed. The "failure to adapt" to military life, a major reason for conscripts escaping military service in the United States, was not acceptable in the Soviet Army.

In the Soviet Union, every citizen fifty-five years old or younger who was physically fit was called to military service. The draft screening procedure centered around a number of local military commissions or commissariats. This commission was comprised of medical doctors, usually internists and neurologists, who examined conscripts and passed on their general physical health. No psychiatrists served on these examining boards, and no psychiatric tests were administered. Interestingly, in the modern Soviet Army, no psychiatrists serve on the conscript examining boards. Whatever psychiatric screening was done was on an ad hoc basis and was accomplished by neurologists whose physiological orientation permitted them to detect any organic causes that might be responsible for behavioral problems. Those allowed to escape military service for other than clear physical disabilities were those who suffered from imbecillia or who were so obviously psychotic that there was no practical problem in diagnosing them as such. The number of conscripts who were deferred from military service on purely psychiatric grounds was very small indeed. Problems of neurosis were simply not regarded as serious enough to merit exemption and are not regarded as serious enough to defer a Soviet conscript today. Rejections for psychiatric reasons were simply not a major cause of military manpower loss to the Soviets in World War II. Indeed, during the darkest days at the beginning of the war, there was often no time to examine or to validate a soldier's symptoms, and, with no psychiatric tests used at all, the Soviets simply used reasonable medical standards of physical infirmity as a guide for rejection. Those who were clearly too old or infirm were not accepted; everyone else was. It must be remembered, too, that even the physical standards of fitness for military service in the Soviet Union were far lower in World War II than in the West. Since then, of course, the Soviets have used the DOSAAF (the Voluntary Society for Assistance to the Army, Aviation, and Navy of the USSR) system of premilitary training and selection to raise both the general health and enlistment standards of the Soviet conscript.

It is somewhat easier to obtain data on the number of rejections for psychiatric reasons allowed by the Soviets in World War II. To be sure, the data are not definitive. They were obtained by interviewing medical doctors and neurologists who served on draft medical commissions during the war; some even served as battle surgeons later on. According to these sources, of the 22 million men who were conscripted perhaps no more than 50,000 to 75,000 were exempted from military service for purely psychiatric problems. This constitutes a rejection rate of less than 0.25 percent; even at the extreme the figure would not exceed 1 percent of the total pool examined. By comparison, the United States examined some 18 million men and rejected 5,250,000, or about 29 percent of the total pool, for "mental, moral, and physical" reasons. The United States found 71 percent of its conscript pool fit for military duty, or approximately 12,750,000 men. It rejected 970,000 men for neuropsychiatric disorders and other emotional problems. Thus, psychiatric reasons accounted for 18.5 percent of those rejected for military service. As a percentage of the total conscript pool, 5.4 percent of those initially screened for military service were rejected for psychiatric disorders.[17] The rejection rate for psychiatric problems was twenty times greater than in the Soviet Army in World War II.

It might be expected that a substantial number of conscripts would have been rejected for physical reasons largely as a consequence of improper nutrition. This situation was chronic in almost all Western armies in World War I and, in fact, was the primary stimulus for child nutrition programs established in the West after 1918. Between 1920 and 1940, the Soviet Union suffered enormous social disruptions, wars, domestic purges, and even a famine which might have been expected to affect the nutritional quality of the Soviet diet with a concomitant decline in physical health. Yet, Soviet doctors who served on medical examining boards point out that few individuals were exempted from military service because of improper nutritional development. Moreover, it was assumed that in time of war the military would have first call on available food supplies, so that even if one was marginal by nutritional standards, it was assumed that he would be better fed in the military than as a civilian, an assumption that generally proved correct. Unlike the U.S. conscripts who were not physically "fit for battle," they were conscripted anyway and were assigned to noncombat jobs such as cooks, clerks, and medical orderlies. In short, the physical standards of acceptance in the Soviet Army were considerably below those of most armies of the West. The practical result was that the Soviets had far less manpower loss for both physical and psychiatric reasons in the initial selection process than did the United States and most other Western armies.

In attempting to determine the Soviets' effectiveness in reducing the loss of soldiers to neuropsychiatric breakdown, it must be kept in mind that the degree to which military units will generate neuropsychiatric casualties in the first place depends on many variables, not all of which are directly quantifiable (unit cohesion, quality of leadership, replacement system, and so on). Three major factors that are directly quantifiable are the type of battle a unit must fight, its intensity, and its duration. In this regard, the Soviets fought almost five long years of war, much of it under conditions of disarray and near collapse. The intensity of combat, and the size and duration of the battles they fought, were, on balance, much greater than those fought by American and British troops, with the possible exception of the Normandy invasion and the battle for Normandy in July 1944. The Soviet Army suffered more physical casualties than any other combatant, perhaps as many as 8 million dead and another 15 million wounded. World War II was therefore a war of much greater intensity for the Soviets than for most other combatants, with the possible exception of the Germans. On these grounds alone, Soviet military units could be expected to have suffered very high numbers of neuropsychiatric casualties.

In addition, the number of Soviet Army psychiatric casualties can be related to the manner in which they conducted battle. In his study based on an analysis of hundreds of Soviet combat unit histories and diaries, Glantz concludes that it was very common for Soviet divisions to enter battle at only 70 percent strength in manpower and equipment. It was also quite common practice to fight these units down to 25 percent and 30 percent strength before stopping the attack.[18] Even then, Soviet units were often not pulled out of the line. Instead, another division would be thrown into the breach, joining the remaining elements of the bloodied unit to the new one, and continuing the attack. These practices suggest that the tempo of war was very intense for Soviet units and that Soviet battle doctrine itself probably increased what was an already high level of combat dead, wounded, and stress casualties. By comparison, American divisions almost never went into battle without an overage of combat strength in manpower and equipment; it was common practice to enter battle at greater than 100 percent strength. Furthermore, the Americans would fight a unit down to only 70 percent strength. Even today, any American battle unit that suffers 30 percent casualties is no longer considered to be combat effective. In World War II, units that suffered 30 percent casualties were almost always pulled from the line and rotated to the rear for replenishment of men and equipment. These figures suggest that Soviet battlefield practice was likely to engender a much greater level of stress and concomitant psychiatric casualties among units than did Western battlefield practice.

The propensity to fight units down to the nub before replacing them contributed strongly to the Soviets' level of psychiatric casualties. Forcing depleted units to join new units and continue the attack only made matters worse and increased psychiatric casualties. The tendency was to continue the attack until the objective was seized; only then was rest and replenishment likely to occur. The mode of fighting was far less like a gradual streamroller, an analogy often used in Western military commentaries, than it was like a giant, irresistible, but short-lived pulse. The Soviets displayed a tendency to engage in long periods of rest and replenishment before a battle, building their forces and positioning them for the attack. Once the attack began, it was carried out with great violence, often from the front, and continued until the objective was secured or until the attacking forces collapsed from exhaustion or decimation. The Soviets appeared willing to accept staggering numbers of casualties in the pursuit of military objectives, something that often led Western, particularly German, generals to disregard the abilities of Soviet high-level commanders. A good example of all these tactical characteristics was Operation Little Saturn , an offensive against the Italian Army after the battle of Stalingrad. True to form, Soviet units entered battle at 70 percent strength, fought down to 25 percent strength as they took horrendous losses, but continued the offensive until they broke the defender's back.

When the circumstances of battle or an army's fighting doctrine increase the number of dead and wounded suffered by military units, the ability of these units to cohere under stress is brought into serious question. Furthermore, inasmuch as the rate of psychiatric casualties generated by units is clearly related to the intensity, duration, and type of battle, and it tends to vary directly with the number of killed and wounded suffered by a unit, Soviet units in World War II probably suffered very high rates of neuropsychiatric casualties. The fact is, however, that the Soviets' rate of psychiatric casualties is not known. There are simply no data available. As we will see, it is possible to determine how many soldiers were lost to units as a result of such casualties. One can point out, however, that American military units often suffered very high rates of psychiatric casualties, and, in many instances, psychiatric casualties exceeded the number of wounded and killed. Because these rates were encountered by American units that generally fought under much less harsh conditions and in battles of less intensity and duration than those of most Soviet units, the rates of initial psychiatric breakdown in Soviet units was likely at least as high as in the American Army and, in all probability, much higher.

The practical challenge of military psychiatry is not how to prevent psychiatric breakdown among men engaged in battle, for, indeed, there is widespread agreement that, whereas the rates of breakdown may be somewhat controllable, the mechanisms that produce psychiatric breakdown in battle are still far beyond the control of psychiatrists. Some psychiatric casualties are inevitable under the horrors of modern war. The more important question for military psychiatry in any army is how effectively does it deal with the numbers of psychiatric casualties that will inevitably result from battle. The practical task of military psychiatry is to treat as many psychiatric casualties as quickly as possible and to return them to their fighting units in order to preserve the manpower strength of an army engaged in warfare. The most significant overall test of military psychiatry, the cultural values of the various combatants aside, is the degree to which it is successful in stopping or reducing manpower loss to fighting units. By this standard, Soviet military psychiatry seems to have done very well during World War II.

As discussed earlier, in World War II, the Soviet Army mobilized approximately 22 million men, of whom 5 million were killed and another 9 million wounded. This means that at least 14 million men saw direct combat, although the figure is realistically higher. Given the nature of the war, fought to a great degree on the Russian homeland, it is possible that as many as 20 million Soviet soldiers faced hostile fire. Drawing on more than a score of interviews with Soviet combat doctors, including psychiatrists and neurologists, we can arrive at a rough estimate of the number of Soviet soldiers who were diagnosed as suffering from psychiatric problems serious enough to warrant evacuation from their units. These men were lost to Soviet combat units for much, if not most, of the war. The data suggest that the loss rate due to neuropsychiatric reasons suffered by the Red Army was certainly under 10 per 1,000 and, probably, closer to 6 per 1,000. This is about the same rate suffered by the American Army in World War I. Using this figure as a baseline, during World War II the Soviet Army suffered between 96,000 and 100,000 psychiatric casualties that were eventually lost to the fighting units as manpower assets.

A comparison can be made between the Soviet Army and the American Army in the same war. If the rate of manpower loss suffered by the American Army for purely psychiatric reasons is examined, it seems that the American Army was less successful in preventing manpower loss to psychiatric breakdown. In the American Army alone (not counting Army air crews, naval or Marine casualties), the United States suffered 504,000 separations from military service as a result of psychiatric problems. Of these, 333,000 were true neuropsychiatric cases of psychosis and psychoneurosis. The difference between the two figures, 171,000, is attributable to separations from service due to "behavioral problems" and the "failure to adapt" to military life.[19] Only 42 percent of all separations effected for psychiatric reasons in the American forces occurred among men who actually faced the enemy. Amazingly, 58 percent of the psychiatric separations occurred in the zone of interior, that is, in the United States before these men were ever sent overseas or into battle![20]

Of the 333,000 separations due to psychosis and psychoneurosis that occurred in combat zones, among those soldiers who saw ground combat duty in Europe, the rate of psychiatric casualty loss was 38 per 1,000. This means that the ground combat army suffered approximately 12,616 neuropsychiatric casualties that were severe enough to be removed from the combat pool for the duration of the war. This figure does not include the thousands that broke down in battle, were treated, and eventually returned to their units. During World War II, approximately 40 percent of the soldiers who suffered psychiatric breakdown were successfully returned to their units.[21] If one examines the ratio of psychiatric casualties to the number of dead and wounded, American ground forces suffered 234,874 dead and 568,861 men wounded. Thus, the ratio of psychiatric casualties to wounded was one to nineteen and the ratio of psychiatric casualties to killed in action was one to forty-three.

These figures suggest that the Soviet Army suffered higher initial rates of psychiatric casualties (certainly they suffered a higher absolute number of such casualties) than did the American Army. Once these casualties occurred, however, the Soviet medical system was able to minimize the rate of manpower loss to fighting units by treating psychiatric patients and keeping them on the front lines. If the overall rates of return are examined, then it is clear that the loss rate due to psychiatric casualties in the American Army was four to six times higher than that in the Soviet Army. Moreover, the ratio of psychiatric casualties to dead was 2.5 times higher than in the Soviet Army, whereas the rate of psychiatric casualties to wounded was twice as high. None of this is to criticize the way in which the American Army dealt with its own psychiatric casualties. But it is to point out that although the Soviets probably suffered a much greater rate of initial psychiatric casualties, they were more successful in containing the eventual manpower loss that could have resulted from these rates. The Soviets were simply able to keep more men fighting more of the time under greater degrees of battle stress than was the American Army in World War II.

3
Soviet Combat Psychiatry in World War II

What policies, doctrines, and practices helped the Soviet Army during World War II to sustain its manpower strength by keeping psychiatric casualty losses to a minimum? One important factor was the manner in which the Soviets perceived the causes of battleshock and the ways in which they were prepared to deal with it. It is a fact of psychiatric life that expectations tend very much to condition behavior. To the extent that certain physical or psychiatric symptoms are regarded as legitimate, when soldiers are placed in situations of extreme stress they will tend to manifest these very symptoms. In this sense, then, the behavioral expectations of the military system have their effect on the soldier, who will then tend to realize these expectations as a way of escaping stressful battlefield situations.

Soviet soldiers who exhibited certain battleshock symptoms were regarded as making a very functional adjustment to their environment. Soldiers who wished to escape the horrors of the battlefield were regarded as essentially normal and sane people who were prepared to go to great lengths to escape their environment. The consequence was that the values of the Soviet military subculture functionally defined what types of behavior it would permit. These values, in turn, framed a set of expectations for both the controllers of the military subsystem and its participants, namely, the soldiers.

Once the subculture defined the legitimate excuses for avoiding battle, then the soldiers were expected to adapt to these standards. Put another way, if a military subculture takes a lenient view of the circumstances a soldier can use to escape the rigors of the battlefield, then the subculture will likely generate higher rates of psychiatric casualties than stricter military systems. In the Soviet case, as one might expect of a totalitarian and ideologically motivated military system, the Soviet view of battleshock was extremely harsh.

The term for "shock" in the Soviet lexicon is "shock," which is equivalent to the Russian *udar*, the same word used to describe a heart attack, epileptic stroke, or even an electrical shock. There is no clinical term for "battleshock." The Soviets use the term "reaction" for psychological symptoms with no accompanying physical cause. They regard such reactions as problems of small psychiatry. The Russian term for shock delineates a condition that is physiologically caused, has physiological symptoms, and is subject to physiological cure. The Soviet view does not admit of a condition of psychiatric breakdown that is induced as a consequence of purely emotional and psychological factors for which there is no accompanying physiological cause. Even in the diagnosis of schizophrenia and severe psychosis, Soviet biological psychiatry places the eventual cause for such diseases in some organic disruption of the brain. In World War II, the Soviets did not regard emotional trauma per se as a legitimate excuse for permitting the soldier relief from battle. The only legitimate excuse allowed the soldier suffering from stress was a symptomology that had a clearly discernible physiological cause due to injury.

Combat shock, according to the Soviets, is organically caused and, therefore, may be corrected by treating the damaged or disrupted physiology of the patient. Those purely emotional or psychic causes which, in the United States, would be regarded as expected consequences of battlefield stress, are viewed by Soviet psychiatrists as manifest shortcomings in the soldier's character, motivation, or training. The fact that a soldier may be too frightened to move, suffer tremors, have difficulty processing information, be reluctant to fire his weapon, or any number of other symptoms is not taken seriously. They regard such conditions as normal battlefield conditions and place the responsibility for dealing with them and continuing to function squarely on the soldier.

As observed earlier, the Soviets regard a soldier who suffers abnormally high levels of anxiety, fear, or panic as an individual who either has a defect in his character or is suffering from problems of improper motivation, morale, and training. They blame failures of morale and motivation not only on the soldier, but also on the unit commander and, most particularly, on the political officer. Normal symptoms of battle stress are not seen as a medical problem; indeed, except for psychosis, all neurosis among combat soldiers is defined as a nonmedical problem.

In World War II, the Soviets refused to admit that a whole range of psychiatric casualties were, in fact, psychiatric casualties at all. Instead of treating them in the medical and evacuation chain, they were simply turned over to unit commanders and political officers to be dealt with on a motivational basis. Intriguingly, this refusal to treat as a medical problem what in other armies were regarded as legitimate maladies, and to deal with them as command and administrative problems at the small-unit level, seems to have considerably reduced the rate of neuropsychiatric casualties suffered by the Red Army. The Soviets were, therefore, able to avoid the large-scale evacuation of soldiers with these symptoms and to hold them in the battle zone much longer. Only physically based symptoms or cases of obvious psychosis were taken seriously as medical problems; all other manifestations were regarded as problems of small psychiatry.

Soviet psychiatrists distinguished between what they called big psychiatry and small psychiatry in attempting to diagnose psychiatric problems. Problems of big psychiatry referred to illnesses associated with organic disorders or disruptions of the brain, and tended largely to focus on schizophrenia and the other major psychoses. These behavioral manifestations could be traced to organic injuries caused largely by some sort of commotion, concussion, or contusion leading to organic brain damage, including neurologic injuries to the spinal cord. Almost all other symptoms evident in combat soldiers—fear, anxiety, tremors, inability to sleep, partial paralysis, and a range of other symptoms—were regarded as problems of small psychiatry normally diagnosed in a range of temporary to permanent neurosis. Problems of small psychiatry were left to unit commanders, political officers, and, in more severe cases, to neurologists.

In the opinion of many Soviet psychiatrists and other physicians who served in World War II, unit commanders and political officers became excellent clinical diagnosticians in their ability to separate the truly serious cases of psychosis and other problems due to organic damage from less serious problems. Colonel Glantz, in his study of Soviet units in World War II, notes that the role of the political officer in motivating soldiers to fight well has been grossly underestimated and distorted in the military histories of the West. He points out that the political officer was often the focal point of the unit in terms of sustaining morale and motivation.[1]

Each battalion had a political officer who was charged with ensuring the motivation, morale, and fighting spirit of his unit. At the battalion level, the political officer often had a small staff that went down into the companies and carried out similar tasks. When soldiers failed to demonstrate the proper motivation and morale, failed to perform correctly, or began to show symptoms normally associated with combat stress, Soviet units assigned a political officer to deal immediately with the problem. The presence of this officer within the unit accompanied by a comparatively harsh doctrine as to what symptoms qualified as a legitimate reason to evacuate a soldier from the front led the Soviets to apply two of the basic principles of combat psychiatry, namely, expectancy and proximity of treatment. These two principles applied most directly to the range of problems associated with small psychiatry. The result was a low rate of manpower loss to combat units due to psychiatric problems.

Although severe by U.S. standards, undeniably the Soviet system worked very well. Any soldier with psychiatric symptoms who came to the attention of the medical officer or feldsher at battalion level, but who manifested no accompanying physical problem, was regarded with suspicion. These patients were regarded as soldiers attempting to escape combat and were treated as such. Many of the men who had purely psychiatric symptoms were handled by the unit commander, the political officer, or the battalion feldsher and then forced to return to their units. A common method of dealing with these soldiers was to give them a severe tongue lashing, have his peers talk to him and convince him to return, or even threaten the soldier with assignment to a penal battalion. In extreme cases, threats of execution were used and sometimes carried out. Soviet battlefield discipline in World War II was severe, and the execution of a soldier who failed to perform was viewed as merely company punishment that required no trial or hearing and from which there was no appeal. To be sure, this approach could not be used too frequently without an officer risking retaliation from the soldier's comrades often in the form of shooting the officer! In interviewing Soviet veterans of World War II, one is impressed by the number of respondents who say they recall instances in their own units where officers and NCOs were shot by their own men. When such assassinations occurred, those who were responsible were most often not executed themselves but were assigned to penal battalions.

In any event, there were enough battlefield executions of soldiers who would not perform adequately to give credence to the threat. And if one was not shot, there was always the possibility that a soldier would be sent to a penal battalion where he would endure a much harsher life with a greater chance of being killed than even at the front line. Assignments to penal battalions meant certain combat under the most difficult and often suicidal conditions. Common practice was to force penal battalions to fight in the snow without camouflaged uniforms or to march them across minefields in order to clear the way for advancing units. In the United States, of course, assignment to a penal battalion meant escape from combat. Although one lived under harsh prison conditions, one was at least free from the terrors of the battlefield.

Soviet military psychiatry in World War II used a strict definition of the "ticket out," the set of symptoms that was required before a soldier was allowed to be evacuated from the front lines. The Soviet ticket was defined in nonpsychic, almost purely neurological terms in that it required some physical cause—commotion, contusion, concussion, or other traumatic injury to the brain or spinal cord—that could be reasonably assessed as causing the soldier's behavioral problem. Not only did the Soviets require that the cause of the problem be organically based, but, most often, the diagnostic screen also required that the behavioral symptomology be accompanied by a physiological effect such as paralysis, bleeding from the ears or nose, hysteria, or surdomutism. Soldiers who came to the attention of medical personnel but who lacked these physiological elements of diagnosis were regarded as shirkers and cowards to be dealt with as such.

Given the assumption that a soldier's problems were organically caused and were accompanied by distinct physical symptoms that could be traced to this damage, Soviet medical personnel assumed that both symptoms and causes could be treated much more readily than was generally the case in the United States. The Soviets—no doubt remembering their experience in the Russo-Japanese War and World War I—assumed from the beginning that the organic causes of psychiatric problems required rapid treatment close to the battlefront. Wherever the soldier with a true psychiatric problem was treated—at division, army, or front level—the task was to treat the physical injury and return the soldier as rapidly as possible to the battlefield. Thus, Soviet combat psychiatry in World War II was based not only on the principles of proximity and expectancy, but also on the third principle of military psychiatry, immediacy of treatment. Because the causes of psychiatric debilitation were seen to be traceable to organic injury, Soviet treatment tended to stress physical methodologies. As a result, Soviet psychiatrists could avoid dealing with the soldier's psyche and other emotional problems, and could deal directly with the soldier's body and brain. This made the provision of treatment close to the front comparatively easy and more rapid and, in fact, seems to have increased the probability of recovery.

Both medical and command personnel had high expectations that soldiers suffering psychiatric problems would be returned to the battlefront as quickly as possible. When the rate of psychiatric breakdown reached such proportions as to begin to affect whole units, these units were immediately dealt with by special police units and investigators. A high rate of psychiatric casualties in a unit was attributable to a failure on the part of the commander and the political officer. Units that did not perform well in battle came in for severe action from special police units. At times whole units were imprisoned and their leaders were executed in full view of their men. Harsh as it may seem, the expectation on the part of commanders and Soviet medical personnel that psychiatric cases were not to be taken seriously, to be dealt with immediately and, if this failed, to be dealt with harshly, had the desired effect of reducing manpower loss as a consequence of psychiatric casualty rates. What were the long-term effects of these policies on soldiers who suffered psychiatric symptoms once they left the military and returned to civilian life, and how many suffered a post-traumatic stress reaction? These are questions that must be left unanswered.

The Soviet medical system for dealing with psychiatric casualties set a high and diagnostically precise price for excusing a soldier from battle. As noted earlier, the Soviets considered many of the reasons allowed in Western armies as simply a soldier's normal reactions in battle and defined them as insufficient to relieve the soldier from the fighting. Soldiers suffering from severe stress symptoms might be granted a short period of rest at the battalion or regimental aid station. But, in general, their symptoms were not regarded as sufficient cause to evacuate them further to the rear. The Soviet medical evacuation system gave priority to the physically wounded and thus mitigated against the evacuation of psychiatric casualties who did not exhibit some sign of organic damage. For example, a soldier discovered at the regimental aid station to be suffering from paralysis of the legs would be given a cursory physical examination. If no clear organic cause for his paralysis was found, say a bullet wound or other physiological damage, he would be removed from the medical evacuation chain and put aside at the aid station until events quieted down enough for him to be given further attention.

The Soviet medical evacuation system in World War II was extremely primitive, when it existed at all, and could hardly operate in any consistent manner. The initial suspicion with which psychiatric symptoms were met, coupled with few mechanisms for diagnosing psychiatric casualties with no accompanying physical damage, when added to a medical evacuation system that was barely functional, meant that, in practice, fewer psychiatric cases got into the evacuation train to begin with. Certainly far fewer than was the case in the American Army where as a matter of bad habit doctors who could not find any physiological damage on a psychiatric patient normally evacuated him anyway. Because the Soviet medical evacuation system was unable and unwilling to evacuate anyone without serious physical injury, most psychiatric casualties were retained for longer periods within the battle zone where they were treated by unit commanders, political officers, sanitors, feldshers, and regimental surgeons.

As noted earlier, soldiers tend to respond to the expectations and punishments of their military subculture. Soviet soldiers knew unequivocally that without any real physical damage to justify their claim to psychiatric disability their chances of escaping the battlefield were slim, whereas their chances of being severely disciplined or sent to a penal battalion or even shot were considerably greater. These realities obviously conditioned their behavior to a great extent. Moreover, the requirement that psychiatric problems be accompanied by a discernible physical symptom led soldiers to convert their stress reactions into precisely these symptoms.

The Soviets simply had a different set of expectations of their soldiers than did other armies and used a different set of clinical definitions to diagnose legitimate psychiatric problems. By rigorously enforcing these definitions and expectations through stern battlefield discipline, they were able to reduce their manpower loss. None of this says anything about the ability to prevent initial psychiatric breakdown which, as already observed, was probably at least as high in its initial occurrence as in other armies in the West and, given the nature of the battles the Soviet Army had to fight, probably somewhat higher.

The Soviet approach to neuropsychiatric casualties during World War II was reflected in the structure of its medical care and treatment. An analysis of this structure shows a lack of formal psychiatric training among medical personnel below regimental level. Indeed, there were no psychiatrists or psychiatric treatment staff at division level, a condition that was common in Western armies during World War II and that had existed in some armies since World War I. One can legitimately conclude that the Soviet medical structure emphasized the treatment of physiological casualties and that psychiatric casualties were either ignored, given very low priority, or else treated largely as patients whose behavioral problems stemmed from physiological injuries.

At the army and front levels, however, there were special hospitals and staff for dealing with psychiatric patients. Few patients who were not diagnosed as having major psychosis or schizophrenia ever reached these hospitals, however. The great majority of psychiatric cases suffered from problems of small psychiatry and were never evacuated beyond division. At the front level hospital, located about 100 miles to the rear of the fighting, a complete psychiatric hospital and a staff of six to eight psychiatrists and neurologists were often attached to the usual surgical hospital. Psychiatric patients were treated by psychiatrists and neurologists, although once again, the bulk of the treatment seems to have been directed by neurologists focusing on the organic damage that was causing the behavioral problem. The front level hospital had facilities for about 100 psychiatric patients.

Closer to the fighting was the army level hospital, located between fifty and seventy-five miles from the battle. This facility had a small psychiatric ward capable of accommodating forty patients. Yet, only some of these beds were actually set aside for psychiatric patients. The psychiatric staff of the army level hospital consisted of two to three doctors. Sometimes army level hospitals had no psychiatrists at all but relied on neurologists to treat patients. Usually, however, at least one psychiatrist was in residence. This tendency to mix psychiatrists and neurologists, as noted earlier, has a long history in Soviet psychiatric practice and is based on the assumption that behavioral aberrations derive essentially from organic disruptions of the brain and nervous system.

At division level there were no provisions at all for psychiatrists or psychiatric staffs. The division had a basic medical battalion that provided normal casualty treatment support to the division. Below division, there were doctors located at the regimental aid station which supplemented the division aid station. Many of the doctors at regimental level were neurologists, but most were battle surgeons ranging from trained surgeons to general practitioners. Below regiment was the battalion aid station staffed by a feldsher and a few medics and, below this, at company level, one found only the normal complement of company medics. Thus, at division or below, the Soviet Army made no provisions for treating psychiatric casualties. Even when psychiatric casualties reached the division level hospital, by and large they were treated by neurologists and other medical doctors, for no psychiatrists were assigned at this level. As one moved further toward the front, one found fewer and fewer medical personnel of any sort. Furthermore, no effort was made to incorporate in the training of Soviet medical personnel below division any knowledge of combat psychiatry. Nonetheless, those with experience became excellent diagnosticians insofar as they were able to separate problems of big psychiatry from the more normal behavioral problems that occur in all soldiers under stress.

In some other armies, the inability to diagnose psychiatric cases led to the shunting of psychiatric casualties with marginal physical symptoms into the normal medical evacuation chain. As a consequence of either misdiagnosis or ignorance, great numbers of psychiatric casualties who could have easily been retained at the front or within the battle zone were needlessly evacuated from battle. Once in the evacuation chain, it was almost impossible to get out until one was evacuated deeply to the rear. In the Soviet Army, the opposite happened. Being untrained in psychiatric diagnosis, lower level medical personnel tended to reinforce the system's predominant notion that certain behaviors were normal consequences of fear or reflected defects in character. Such patients were kept in the command and administrative chain and diverted, as the system was designed to do, to commissars and unit commanders to be dealt with accordingly.

The Soviet military strongly reinforced this practice by blaming a unit's high rates of psychiatric casualties on a breakdown of command and leadership and placing the responsibility directly on the unit commander. In addition, every battalion and regiment had a political officer who was directly responsible for the morale, motivation, and ideological fighting strength of his unit. High levels of psychiatric casualties were seen as the political officer's failure to do his job. Paradoxically, although the Soviet system did not formally assign psychiatrists and other clinically trained personnel to lower unit levels to aid in the diagnosing and treatment of psychiatric casualties, in practice, the system worked as well as if they did. By charging both the unit commander and the political officer with maintaining the fighting spirit of the unit, the commander and commissar developed a strong personal interest in keeping the rates of evacuation for psychiatric reasons to a minimum. They were forced to deal with such problems on the spot or face the prospect of serious consequences themselves.

Soviet commanders and medical personnel understood, however, that some psychiatric illnesses were so severe that they had to be recognized for what they were, although it was not necessary to admit their etiological derivation. In instances of genuine psychosis, soldiers were evacuated rapidly. In these cases, the feldshers, medics, and battalion surgeons diagnosed the psychotic, separating him from those who were suffering only "normal" combat reactions or problems of small psychiatry. The cases of normal combat reactions were treated as close to their fighting units as possible. At each stage of the evacuation, depending on the seriousness of the problem, psychiatric patients were given lower priority than physical casualties, and they were often left at battalion, regimental, or division aid stations where they were allowed to rest until they could be examined more thoroughly. After a few days of rest, even soldiers with the most severe nonpsychotic combat reactions were usually returned to the fighting. Psychotic individuals, on the other hand, were immediately removed from their fighting units and isolated until they could be evacuated. As they moved further to the rear, at each stage they were isolated until they could be treated. This was done not so much out of a humanitarian concern for the soldier as much as out of the realistic consideration that the psychotic could be enormously disruptive in a fighting unit, either through the contagion of fear or the psychotic's own violent actions. By limiting evacuation to those psychiatric cases with extreme and obvious symptoms, the Soviets were able to keep their manpower loss for psychiatric reasons to a minimum. During World War I, the U.S. Army used a similar definition for evacuating psychiatric casualties and employed much the same evacuation procedure. The rates of manpower loss due to psychiatric causes were about the same, for both the U.S. Army in World War I and the Soviet Army in World War II, approximately 6 to 9 per 1,000. During World War II, when the U.S. Army adopted a more lenient definition of psychiatric casualties, the loss rate skyrocketed to between 36 and 39 per 1,000.

Interviews with a number of Soviet soldiers who served in World War II reveal wide agreement that commanders, feldshers, doctors, and even sanitors were generally able to distinguish problems of big psychiatry from the other symptoms attendant to battle stress. If a soldier was diagnosed as being a psychiatric casualty because of traumatic damage to his brain or neurological system, he was normally not badgered by his commander or political commissar. Such a diagnosis, however, usually had to be made by a psychiatrist or a neurologist. Perhaps this reflects the Russian penchant for bureaucracy. Once an official diagnosis was made, the unit commander and the political officer were off the hook. They could now point to someone else who had taken responsibility for a soldier who would not fight. Even so, commanders and political officers understood that sometimes a soldier could no longer function and, that to continue to threaten and cajole was pointless. In general, psychiatric diagnosis involved some statement that the soldier was suffering from traumatic encephalopathy, namely, organic damage to the brain or neurological system that prevented him from functioning and to which his behavioral symptoms could be traced. But commanders and political officers could be harsh with soldiers whose behavioral problems had no clear organic explanation.

One means which the Soviets used to reduce the level of battleshock casualties was to narrow the diagnostic definition of a neuropsychiatric casualty. Not surprisingly, their treatment of battleshock was a continuation of the biological approach to psychiatry that had been evident in Russia since at least 1860. Psychiatrists sustained the belief that behavioral aberration on the battlefield had a physical cause, usually "brain shock" or, more clinically, traumatic encephalopathy. This implied some sort of brain damage that interfered with proper function. The basic diagnostic assumption was that soldiers suffering from behavioral problems, psychosis, and even neurosis were suffering from organic damage to the brain.

As a major cause of overt behavioral problems, Soviet psychiatrists singled out concussion, commotion, and contusion of the brain, usually associated with loss of consciousness. This focus accurately reflects the terminology used by the French in World War I in their attempts to explain psychiatric reactions to battle stress. In more precise terms, Soviet psychiatrists, being first and foremost medical doctors educated in the Germanic tradition of biological psychiatry, attributed behavioral aberrations to some form of bruising of the brain, microbleeding in the interior of the brain, the presence of brain lesions, edema, and microscopic scars caused by trauma or disease. The approach was to attempt to link the soldier's overt behavioral symptoms—paralysis, mutism, blindness, and so on—to the damage that may have been done to certain areas of the brain. American, German, French and British military psychiatrists used this same diagnostic approach early in World War I but by the Second World War it had largely been abandoned in favor of less strict, less biological, and more psychic and emotional explanations.

Battlefield medical personnel concerned themselves with the organic causes of behavioral aberration and operationally distinguished between neurosis and depression psychosis. Soldiers exhibiting neurosis or small psychiatry symptoms were sent to their unit commanders or other nonmedical personnel for treatment. Psychiatrists focused on depression psychosis, that is, bizarre symptoms and behavior such as curling up into a fetal position or hearing voices or severe conversion syndromes. Battalion and company medical personnel did the screening for these conditions. With unit commanders treating small psychiatry problems and other medical personnel acting essentially as diagnostic screens, who did that leave for combat psychiatrists to treat? Based on interviews with Soviet doctors who served in World War II, Soviet soldiers seem to have suffered a very high rate of conversion reactions. Yet, this situation would not be unexpected. As noted earlier, soldiers respond to those precise symptoms that the system defines as acceptable for escaping battle. With Soviet psychiatrists having defined brain damage causing overt physiological manifestations as the way out of battle, soldiers, of course, began to convert their fears and anxieties into precisely these manifestations. This phenomenon is not unknown in armies generally. Such conversion reactions as hysteria, surdomutism, partial paralysis, and fugue states—all familiar to Western combat psychiatrists—were common.

Soviet neurologists point out that the rate of conversion reactions became so high in the army that doctors and other field medical personnel had to develop shorthand tests to determine which conversion reactions were genuine, which symptoms were tied to organic damage, and which were shallow enough to qualify as faking. Of course, the Soviets immediately rejected any notion that the conversion reactions were produced by purely emotional considerations. Most of these tests were simple and apparently worked quite well. Many were drawn from similar treatments used by the German Army and other Western armies in World War I, and no doubt the Russian Army used a number of them in World War I.

A soldier suffering from a conversion reaction would normally be seen first by a feldsher or medic. The first step was to isolate the patient in a designated area of the battalion or regimental aid station. After a time—usually a few hours—medical personnel would check on him to determine if his conversion state had abated at all or, as in many cases, had disappeared altogether. If the symptoms had lessened, he would be allowed to remain there for up to two days. If a soldier began to come around, he would usually be assigned a task in the aid station area to keep him busy. Much of the time he was simply allowed to rest for twenty-four or thirty-six hours. In the interim, the aid station's medical personnel continued to perform their priority mission, the treatment of the wounded and dying. Once the soldier began to recover, he would be sent back to his unit, or his political officer would come for him. If his symptoms did not abate or grew worse, the soldier was evacuated to regiment.

There were no doctors below the regimental level, and most of those at the regimental level were general medical practitioners and some neurologists. If the soldier was evacuated to regiment, the doctors assumed that his problem had an organic cause. Once a patient suffering severe conversion symptoms reached regiment, the search for the organic origin began. If the doctor suspected that there was no organic cause for the patient's behavior, the soldier would be returned to the regimental aid station and allowed to rest for a few hours or even a few days in order to permit his symptoms to abate. If he began to come around, he would, as at the battalion level, be given some task to perform. A number of Soviet battle surgeons confirm that much of the manpower in the division's medical company—litter bearers, cooks, orderlies, and so on—were often comprised of soldiers who were being held at division while their psychiatric symptoms cleared up. A recovering psychiatric patient could normally function quite well in this role as long as he was kept safe from the direct risks of battle.

After a day or two, the soldier was examined by the regimental surgeon in order to find the organic cause of his symptoms. The practical experiences of war had shown that, despite Soviet psychiatric theory, soldiers were quite capable of sustaining symptoms of organic damage when no such damage was present. For these cases, Soviet medical field personnel administered treatments designed to determine the nature of the patient's illness and to produce counter stimuli that might improve his condition.

One of the most commonly used techniques was the Kaufmann Method, invented by French psychiatrists and used by the German Army in World War I. The test had been developed before World War I in civilian clinical applications and had been taught at Russian medical schools before the war. It was a treatment designed specifically for patients suffering from surdomutism. The object of the treatment was to force the patient to speak as a way of breaking the syndrome. Electrodes were placed on the patient's throat, and moderately intense and painful electrical current was administered. The patient was told that the point of the treatment was to reestablish the damaged pathways from his throat to his brain. In truth, Soviet psychiatrists probably did not believe this. What they were trying to do was to shock the brain, as in electroconvulsive therapy which was also used in other cases, into acting normally again. From the patient's perspective, he had a choice between sustaining his symptoms by enduring a considerable amount of pain or abandoning his symptoms as a way of ridding himself of the pain. This same method was used to treat patients suffering from partial paralysis, a widespread occurrence in Western armies in World War I. The paralysis often took the form of contractive paralysis of the arm needed to operate the bolt of the soldier's weapon. Electric stimulation was administered directly to the affected limb.

Another method used in conversion reactions was to place a rubberized mask over the patient's face and to gradually induce a feeling of suffocation. This technique was used to treat soldiers suffering from fugue states, inability to speak, and paralysis. Again the object was to force the patient to choose between sustaining his symptoms under great discomfort and relinquishing his symptoms by making some physical effort or crying out to remove the mask. The premise behind the test was that only those whose conditions were traceable to organic injury would be able to tolerate the suffocation until they lost consciousness. A variation of the technique was to wrap a rag around the patient's face and pour water on it to simulate the feeling of drowning in the hope that he would respond. Still another test was to poke the paralyzed limbs of the soldier with needles in order to produce enough pain to get him to respond with movement. Not uncommonly, soldiers in fugue states or deep conversion states were able to sustain the pain and discomfort administered. Soldiers in fugue states were often tested by the simple device of making a sudden loud noise and watching for physiological reactions that would prove the state was not induced by true organic damage. Although medical personnel at all levels of the medical treatment system used these tests, they were most frequently employed by doctors at the army and division levels.

Soviet psychiatrists and doctors report that in a large number of cases, especially after the soldier had a few days of rest away from the fighting, these treatments met with success.

The screening methods for holding psychiatric patients at the lower level aid stations and returning them to their units after short periods of rest worked well with most of the small psychiatry problems. Those patients who finally made it to the regimental or division surgeons were subjected to tests and treatments that often worked effectively to eliminate their symptoms. When the patients did not respond, they were examined further to determine the presence of physical damage that could be treated. Even when faced with genuine psychiatric problems, the tendency was not to evacuate a patient beyond division if it could be avoided. The doctors and commanders feared that once a patient was evacuated for purely psychiatric reasons, other soldiers would be encouraged to develop similar symptoms. Thus, every effort was made to find some assignment for the soldier so that he could continue to serve. Even rest was normally accomplished within the general zone of fighting. As noted, many psychiatric patients were assigned as litter bearers, cooks, general helpers, or any number of minor jobs in the division medical company. By keeping soldiers in a useful job, no matter how minor, even broken manpower had some value. Moreover, a soldier assigned a task in the rear area was much more likely to recover than the soldier evacuated further to the rear. Today, both the American and Israeli armies favor placing psychiatric casualties in a military environment and requiring them to do minor tasks as part of a program to prevent any deepening of symptoms and, eventually, to return them to duty.

As in any army, in times of heavy combat, the system broke down. Medical support in the Soviet Army in World War II was primitive to begin with, and, when large numbers of casualties occurred, the system's ability to deal with them declined rapidly. Under these conditions the Soviet Army's treatment of psychiatric casualties differed from that of most Western armies. In the West, for example, when heavy casualties taxed the medical system, soldiers with psychiatric symptoms were often placed in the medical chain and evacuated to the rear rather than being detained and treated at the front. This practice further burdened the entire evacuation and treatment system. When Soviet casualties became heavy, however, those suffering from psychiatric problems were treated even more harshly. In general, if a soldier could walk and had no obvious physical wound, he was immediately turned back to the fighting. In addition, special military police units conducted regular patrols through the medical aid stations, gathering up stragglers or soldiers who were not wounded and forcing them back into the line. As a result, when physical casualties increased, the number of psychiatric evacuations actually decreased—exactly the opposite of what happened in most Western armies.

The Soviets were very successful in returning neuropsychiatric casualties to the fighting. Soldiers showing symptoms traceable to organic injuries were evacuated. But, even here, they were given low priority on the evacuation list. Very often they were left for long periods at designated areas in aid stations until the flow of casualties had subsided. As casualties mounted, the selection criteria for evacuation of psychiatric casualties became even more stringent than normal, with the consequence that fewer psychiatric patients were eventually evacuated.

During World War II, the only soldiers who received serious treatment from psychiatrists were those who were evacuated back to army level hospitals. Those treated at the front were, as noted, treated perfunctorily or, in many cases, not at all and returned quickly to the fighting. Patients who were evacuated to army or front level were those suffering from genuine psychosis or severe conversion reactions; others were so deranged that they could not function. Almost all of these, with some exceptions among the psychotics, manifested some physiological symptoms accompanying whatever battle trauma they had suffered. In other cases, diagnoses indicated cases of deep reactive psychosis. Because the screening procedure operated so effectively, if not very humanely, at the lower levels, only the most severe cases of battleshock were finally evacuated.

The treatments administered at army and front level hospitals were essentially the same as those used by the French, Germans, Americans, and British in World War I for similar cases. A psychiatric casualty sent to an army level hospital had a normal stay of two weeks for mild cases, three weeks for moderate cases, and up to six weeks for the most severe cases. Those who recovered in this time were sent back to the front. For the most part, the Soviets did not make great efforts to return recovered soldiers to their units. The Soviets, aware that their practice of fighting units down to the nub would result in very high casualties to combat units, probably did not see much value in attempting to return soldiers to units which, in many cases, had been decimated or destroyed while the patient was recovering in the hospital. In some instances, Soviet front commanders prohibited sending men back to their units, although a number of Soviet soldiers have reported cases of recovered soldiers fleeing replacement depots in attempts to find comrades in their old units.

The Soviets did not use a unit replacement system during the war, as did the Germans and British, but, instead, adopted an individual replacement system built around replacement depots that strongly resembled the system used by the United States.[2] Soldiers recovering from wounds or combat shock were gathered up by special police units and taken to replacement depots where new units were formed or from which individuals in small groups were sent to units already committed or preparing to go into battle. The special police units would regularly visit the hospitals at the army and front levels, especially the psychiatric hospital wards, in order to ensure the return of every soldier capable of returning to the fighting. Whatever else one may think of the system in terms of its lack of humanity and compassion, it worked very well in reducing manpower loss. When it is recalled that almost every soldier in the Soviet Army who wasn't killed was wounded at least once, this ability to recover the wounded and return them to battle looms large as a factor in the ability of the Soviet Army to achieve victory.

Interviews with Soviet neurologists, psychiatrists, and surgeons who worked at army level hospitals suggest that the Soviets were able to return well over 80 percent of the cases held in psychiatric wards, a figure twice as high as the 40 percent returned by the American Army. The task was made somewhat more difficult by the fact that only the most severe cases of psychiatric debilitation reached the rear in the first place and that the absolute number of psychiatric casualties at all levels of the medical structure was much greater than that in Western armies. Furthermore, the 80 percent who were returned did so within six to eight weeks of being evacuated, a comparably short time to return severe cases of psychiatric debilitation. In institutionalizing mechanisms designed to locate, examine, and return recovered neuropsychiatric casualties to the line, the Soviet Army was practicing a basic principle of military psychiatry, the principle of expectancy. The Soviet soldier expected that no matter what else happened, unless he was so severely wounded that he could no longer function at all, he would be returned to battle. That the medical treatment system returned over 80 percent of its psychiatric cases to the front, and probably at least as high a percentage of those physically wounded, reinforced the Soviet soldier's belief.

With their emphasis on physiological causes of battleshock, not surprisingly the Soviets found that only the most severe psychiatric cases ended up at rear level hospitals. Soviet psychiatrists tended to attribute most combat shock reactions, especially conversion reactions, to brain damage which caused a disruption in the brain's normal functions. Consequently, treatment techniques were most concerned with curing the damage done to the brain and preventing the formation of scar tissues and lesions which they felt could lead to long-term psychiatric problems. Much of the drug and chemical treatment provided by psychiatrists was aimed at preventing scar tissue, reducing edema, and healing lesions.

Diagnostically, the Soviets reported some severe conversion reactions which Western armies also witnessed in World War I: severe hysteria, surdomutism, paralysis, blindness, and others. They also encountered severe depression psychosis sometimes accompanied by memory loss, schizophasia, severe tremors and convulsions, and inability to control bodily functions. Because the Soviet "ticket out" was defined in physiological terms, most of the symptomology emerged in these terms. The highest rates of psychiatric casualties were found among infantrymen, and the second highest among soldiers in the armored corps.[3] Soviet psychiatrists did not find this unusual, for infantrymen were often subjected to artillery bombardments that caused contusions and concussions. Armored troops were often banged around inside their machines and lost consciousness. At army level hospitals, soldiers who did not recover after six weeks were sent rearward to the front level hospitals where the same time schedule for recovery used at the army level hospital obtained. Generally, few psychiatric casualties recovered at front level, and most were placed in the civilian public health system (such as it was!) where they were normally discharged from the military.

Treatment of neuropsychiatric casualties at army and front level hospitals involved significant use of drugs. Perhaps the term "drugs" is an inadequate term if by drugs one means relatively sophisticated chemical agents which can be used to treat specific brain disorders with some precision. More correctly, Soviet psychiatrists relied on a range of plant and animal derivatives that were in the category of folk medicines. To be sure, authentic drugs such as chloryl hydrate and barbiturates were also used, but during World War II no army had sophisticated drugs for the treatment of psychiatric problems.

With this caveat, one can still point to a range of folk medicines, usually plant and animal derivatives, that Soviet psychiatrists found helpful in dealing with battleshock cases. With their belief in the physiological origin of psychiatric disruption, the use of chemical compounds to treat brain damage made good sense. A common treatment, also found in the West, required the administration of chloryl hydrate to induce long periods of sleep as part of general rest therapy. Early in the war, Soviet psychiatrists, as did many psychiatrists in other armies, learned that even the most severe manifestations of combat shock, including reactive psychosis, would often respond well to a period of concentrated sleep. To induce sleep, chloryl hydrate drops were frequently used. The results were often dramatic and rapid.

Another treatment involved the use of what Soviet physicians called brom or bromide, which was also used in the United States at that time. It took the form of either natrium bromide or sodium bromide administered intravenously. It calmed the patient down and put him into a shallow sedative state. The drug was also widely used to build up body fluids and to treat brain concussions, contusions, and seizures. Bromide use was discontinued in the United States when it was found to cause brain damage. Bromide in intravenous form in the Soviet Army may well have been one of those general analgesic therapies that owed as much of its success to the fact that the patient perceived that he was receiving some sophisticated treatment as to the actual therapeutic effect of the compound itself.

Other herb medicine compounds used by Soviet psychiatrists

included valeriana or valadium, ginseng, powdered reindeer horn, goldroot, and mandarin root, all of which were sedatives or stimulants. The Soviets made extensive use of aloe in liquid form administered intravenously. In the United States aloe has recently been used in suntan lotion and in medications for insect bites and minor burns. The Soviets found that it was useful in treating a range of traumatic brain injuries and that it was a good treatment for preventing the formation of scar tissue in the brain after concussions and contusions. Doctors reported that an excellent treatment for preventing and treating small brain lesions was a compound called "fibs." This natural compound was made from special mud, refined to a liquid and injected subcutaneously. Unfortunately, none of the respondents interviewed were able to provide additional data on its composition or method of manufacture.

Two other treatments were magnesium and calcium chloride administered intravenously. Magnesium was administered intravenously as a sedative and was also useful in combating brain edema. The dosage could be controlled for long periods of time, inducing a sedative effect on the patient without disrupting too much of the body's chemistry. Calcium chloride was used as a general stimulant. Administered in intravenous form, it was used to gradually raise the patient's excitation level without inducing shock. This treatment was used extensively for stupor, fugue states, neurasthenia, or cases in which patients could not be brought back to full consciousness.

Two treatments used extensively in the United States, narcohypnosis and abreaction, were used only rarely in the Soviet military. Soviet psychiatrists report that they felt that these techniques usually took too long to work, when they worked at all. They also found that patients tended to resist them. The Soviets did use regular hypnosis from time to time, coupled with various tricks, such as telling a patient under hypnosis to eat onions. But in general such techniques were not seen as particularly valuable and were used to determine if the patient was so deeply psychotic that normal short-term therapy would not work. It also seems plausible that narcohypnosis and abreaction were rejected on the grounds that both were essentially techniques based on Freudian assumptions and had no real basis in biological psychiatry. One gets the impression that hypnosis was used only to determine if the patient was faking his symptoms.

After treatment at the army and front level hospitals, those who did not recover (about 20 percent) were shipped further to the rear; they were taken out of the military evacuation chain and seconded to the civilian district health hospitals. There they were separated into two types of cases: the severely psychotic who were not expected to recover, and the moderately psychotic. The first were shipped to mental wards where they were quickly forgotten, and the second were sent to chronic care hospitals. The military operated a small number of special hospitals after the war to treat specific disabilities, but such hospitals were few. All of northwest Russia had only one hospital, a facility located on an island near Leningrad called Valaam. The building complex on the island formerly housed a monastery, but was converted into a military hospital. This hospital had a special psychiatric section with probably fewer than 100 beds. Severe psychiatric cases were normally discharged into the public health system which itself was in shambles. Interviews with Soviet citizens reveal that after the war it was not uncommon to see mentally ill soldiers roaming the streets of cities and villages in considerable numbers, forced to make their way in society as best they could.

Those soldiers who after the war claimed disability pensions for psychiatric problems that could not be traced to physical injuries were generally denied any pensions or help. In order for a Soviet soldier to qualify for a war-connected disability, he had to have a complete medical record justifying his condition. With regard to psychiatric cases, they had to have a certificate signed by a psychiatrist certifying that their condition was due to some brain or neurological injury incurred in battle. If no organic damage could be demonstrated and the soldier was neurotic or even profoundly neurotic, he would be denied a pension. Those who went to the public health system to obtain these certificates often had to face a battery of unpleasant tests to confirm the diagnosis. In many instances, the tests were painful enough to discourage the applicant.

Soviet military psychiatry remained much the same from 1945 to 1967 when it received a renewed emphasis from the military interested in matching the West's progress in the field. Immediately after the war, Soviet military medical personnel conducted a thorough review of their medical experiences during the war and published it in a multi-volume work. A complete volume was prepared on the subject of military psychiatry. By 1967, Soviet military psychiatrists seemed to have realized that the problems of small psychiatry probably needed more study, especially in light of the military's wish to develop a doctrine of preventing combat shock in the new environment of the nuclear battlefield. After the war several psychiatrists and, after 1967, some psychologists received grants from the military to study the problems of small psychiatry as related to battle stress.

The Soviet Army's interest in battleshock again increased after 1967 in response to its studies of war in a nuclear environment in which the level of shock casualties would be enormous. Nonetheless, as of this writing, most of these efforts have been conducted by psychiatrists more than psychologists and have been limited to research settings. What few applications there are have been directed at pilots, submariners, astronauts, and other highly skilled technicians in an effort to control fear and anxiety and prevent degradation of performance. With regard to military psychiatry in the ground combat forces, the World War II experiences have conveyed the message to the military medical establishment that their mechanisms of diagnosis and treatment worked adequately. They have, of course, tried to keep abreast of more modern methods of treatment, especially the revolution in psychopharmacology which began in France in the 1950s, and have attempted to incorporate some of these developments into their own treatment methodologies.

On balance, the Soviets regard their experience with military psychiatry in World War II as superior to the Western experience. The Soviets continue to believe that a strict definition of what constitutes an acceptable level of traumatic stress can itself be very useful in preventing large numbers of psychiatric casualties. As in World War II, this doctrine is still strongly enforced by unit commanders, political officers, and a medical establishment that refuses to recognize psychiatric debilitation, except at the extremes, which is not tied to physical injury. The Soviet system of treating psychiatric casualties is based on the same practical principles of proximity, immediacy, and expectancy that underpin Western military psychiatry. The Soviets regard their experience with psychiatric breakdown as largely a success. They have continued to build on this success and to develop their approach to combat psychiatry from World War II to the present.

4
Modern Soviet Military Psychiatric Theory

The military and political establishments of the Soviet Union developed conjointly, with the political becoming the predominant influence in shaping the military structure. The political leadership attempts to control all aspects of human behavior as they relate to social obedience and conformity. In addition, the Soviet state is organized around a single ideology that purports to explain all aspects of human history and behavior and, perhaps most important, the future development of humankind. The West does not generally appreciate how thorough and compelling all aspects of life are penetrated by Marxist ideology and its concomitant mechanisms of social control. Ideology is of paramount importance in the USSR, for it justifies the regime and the continuation of the oppressive mechanisms of social control. Thus, military psychiatry, like other aspects of social and intellectual life in the Soviet Union, must accommodate and reflect the dominant values, precepts, and assumptions of Marxist-Leninist ideology. Otherwise, military psychiatry would not be allowed to exist.

The methodologies for diagnosing and treating psychiatric disorders, including battleshock, are necessarily based on the state's assumptions and premises regarding human action. Soviet treatment of battleshock cannot be explained without an understanding of how Soviet military psychiatry defines the human psyche, the sources of emotion, the power of the will, and other precepts that touch on human action. The assumptions made about human behavior actually affect human action. If, for example, mental aberration were assumed to be caused by devils, it would not be surprising to find therapies related to exorcism. Nor would it be surprising to discover that those suffering from mental disruption come to display precisely those symptoms that the exorcist can deal with directly. So it is with military psychiatry. If mental breakdown is defined as being due to organic disturbances of the brain or neurological system, then those soldiers who succumb to battleshock are expected to exhibit symptoms indicating organic disruption, say paralysis or mutism. Thus, to understand Soviet military psychiatry we must first understand their epistemology of the psyche—the assumptions about human action and psychic activity that underpin Soviet diagnostic and treatment methodologies. Chief among these assumptions is, of course, the way Marxism sees human nature and human action. Of particular importance to the development and practice of Soviet psychiatry are the materialist aspects of the Marxist dialectic. Accordingly,

dialectical materialism recognizes only one source for everything; matter, while the spiritual or mental is viewed as secondary or derivative from it. The psyche is a property not of any matter, but a particular organized matter, that is, a property of the brain. The brain is the organizer of mental life, the carrier of thoughts, feelings and will. The psyche, as a particular property of highly organized matter and a function of the brain, consistently reflects the objects and phenomena of the real world. Sensations, concepts and thoughts are subjective images of the objective world. The Leninist understanding of the essence of the psyche as a process of reflection is in opposition to the idealistic views (the psyche as divorced from the brain) and the vulgar materialistic ones (the psyche as an outgrowth of the brain) concerning mental phenomena.[1]

For Soviet psychiatrists, consciousness resides in a physiological brain function and is a product of those circumstances found in objective reality. The way people think and react to stimuli, including battle conditions, is a function of their "social historic development." People are, therefore, a product of their environment. Consequently, "the human psyche is a particular property of the brain and its function consists in its ability to reflect objective social reality; it is a product of social historical development and the result of conditions of labor activities and human conduct."[2] Hence, Marxist psychiatry is "rational psychiatry" in that human action flows only and always from conscious thought. It rejects the "irrational" aspects of Western psychiatric thought which hold that some thought and action flow from the subconscious or unconscious.

Soviet psychiatry, as we have seen, focuses on the organic causes of human action and the physiological activity associated with brain activity. Human action is always seen as rational and conscious. By dismissing the unconscious or subconscious as a producer of action, or by defining it as a pathological defect in human character, Soviet psychiatrists place full responsibility for human action on the individual. This is also true for actions that occur under extremely difficult conditions, such as on the battlefield. Western notions that a soldier's behavior under stress can sometimes be attributed to subconscious, unconscious, or even unstoppable drives is rejected as unscientific.

Soviet psychiatry is built around the Marxist-Leninist concept of scientific dialectical materialism as applied to the material aspects of the internal or phenomenological self. The assumption is that the material world exists outside and independently of human beings and that the internal self is a reflection of objective reality expressed in conscious thought and action. People know, reflect, and adapt to an objective reality. This perception allows them to change objective conditions when their needs warrant, and, in this sense, human beings are seen to be infinitely malleable. They can literally change their nature because that nature is but a reflection of objective conditions; changes in these conditions lead to changes in human nature. Accordingly, the basis for conditioning the individual to conform to his or her objective reality is always present.

When human beings acquire new knowledge, their habits and mental states change. This produces a qualitative change in the sense that it actually affects the nature of the individual. It is this premise, the infinite malleability of the human psyche as a consequence of conditioning and adapting to changing objective conditions, that rests at the psychological base of the Soviets' optimism that they can create a new "socialist man" by changing human nature. For most Western psychologists and psychiatrists, the operative assumption is that human nature cannot be changed. Changes in behavior occur in response to attempts to adjust to changing external conditions (coping), but such changes do nothing to affect the fundamental nature of the human animal. This fundamental difference is reflected in both the theory and practice of Soviet and Western military psychiatry.

There is, however, a rough equivalent of the unconscious in Soviet psychiatric thought insofar as unconscious factors can affect modes of thought or behavior that are important to the actor in the conscious state. In the Soviet view, unconsciousness means those automatic physiological responses, such as basic physiological reflexes, carried out when the individual is not in a conscious state, such as when he or she is asleep or involved in other mental processes not involved in a conscious adaptation to reality (flight). In a narrow sense, then, the Soviets would not entirely deny a role to the unconscious in human activity, but would define it very differently and in narrow physiological terms.

Soviet psychiatrists maintain that consciousness is the dominant factor in all human activity and that human action in all its forms is directly related to brain activity. Accordingly, Soviet psychiatrists do not regard unconscious motivation for conscious behavior as significant in psychiatry and tend to denigrate such views as being bourgeois and idealistic. The common notion in the West that an individual's subconscious or unconscious can induce behavioral changes for which that person is not responsible or aware is rejected as undemonstrable nonsense.

The Soviets believe that consciousness resides in brain physiology. Drawing on Pavlov, Soviet psychiatrists would argue that all behavior and consciousness are merely learned conditioned reflexes that result from the brain's reaction to stimuli or shock provided by the environment. This idea originated in the work of I. M. Sechenev (1829–1905) who developed the reflex theory of the psyche by which "all acts of conscious and unconscious life in terms of their origins" are seen as "simple reflexes."[3] Sechenev identified three components of the reflexes that comprise conscious action: (1) the initial component consisting of the external stimuli and the conversion of those stimuli by sensory organs into the process of nervous stimulation transmitted to the brain; (2) the middle component defined as the central processes in the brain which act to create mental states such as sensations, thoughts, and feelings; and (3) the external or behavioral component which represents the action an individual takes as a consequence of those sensations, thoughts, and feelings.[4] This theory of "reflexology," while it has been modified by the clinical development of Soviet psychiatry, rests at the base of Pavlov's contribution to Soviet psychiatry.

Pavlov tried to demonstrate the validity of the reflex theory of the psyche both experimentally and experientially. The epistemology of Soviet military psychiatry is based on the Pavlovian view of human consciousness as consisting of a series of learned responses gained as the organism (man) attempts to orient itself to an objective reality. This view nicely complements the traditional premises of Russian biological psychiatry which locates the origins of all behavior, normal or deviant, in the physiology of the brain.

The human psyche, therefore, is located in the physiology of the brain. The body has receptors, both internal and external, consisting of nerve cells. Nerve cells have two basic properties, excitability and conductivity, so that, when stimulated, they react and transmit the stimulation to other nerve cells. Sensations are transmitted along nerve fibers to the central nervous system where they reach the analyzer section of the brain which sorts out the various stimuli. These stimuli travel to the mid-brain via the nervous system to the diencephalon which is characterized by stable neuron networks that regulate instinctive, conscious, and emotional reactions to the stimuli received. Located in the cerebral cortex, this section of the brain controls the orthonomic reactions and the psychic processes through the twin functions of excitation and inhibition. The cerebral cortex is the most highly developed part of the central nervous system, often referred to as the higher nervous system, and regulates all other parts of the nervous system. This view developed from Pavlov's so-called principle of reflection which holds that

> an agent from either the body's external or internal world strikes some receptor of the nervous system. This blow in the neurological process is transformed into nerve stimulation. This stimulation runs along the nerve fiber as along a wire to the central nervous system and from there, thanks to the established communications networks, along other fibers leading to the working organs and is transformed in turn into the specific cellular process of that organ. Thus, any agent is characteristically to some body function as cause and effect.[5]

People, therefore, learn through conditioned reflexes which are no more than learned biological patterns of response to stimuli located in the cerebral cortex. Initial stimuli create a "zone of excitement" in the cerebral cortex. With each successive stimulus the brain comes to establish a pattern of reacting to the stimulus as the nerve fibers learn to react. Thus, "the mechanism for developing habits is nothing more than the development of conditioned reflexes."[6]

Soviet psychiatric thought links conditioned reflexes to other conditioned reflexes by what it calls signals. Human beings are equipped with two signal systems, a first and second signal system. Both animals and people have a first signal system, but only humans have a second and "there should be no doubt that the basic laws established in the operations of the primary signal should also govern the secondary system because this function is of the very same nerve tissue."[7] In short, the manner in which each signal system works is physiologically the same, a premise of great importance in defining the role of emotions in human action.

The first signal system consists of neurological patterns which result from temporary ties that arise when receptors are impacted by stimuli. In a simpler sense, people form experiences of the surrounding world based on the stimuli received from that world. In Pavlovian terms, one can teach a dog to salivate by showing him a piece of meat and associating it with the sound of a bell. The sound of the bell sets off a learned pattern of response in the dog's brain which triggers salivation. But this is only the initial stage of conditioning and, in humans, it is insufficient. People possess a second signal system in which stimuli arise not out of external stimuli acting on receptors, but in response to learned signs, words, and other designators. Words, feelings, and commands comprise the second set of signals that trigger previously learned responses. For example, a soldier can react to the command to advance given by a superior; he can also react to internalized signals—to be brave— that he generates himself. It is the word or concept that triggers a pattern of previously learned or conditioned motor activity.

The way individuals learn and observe proper behavior, therefore, is by first developing physiological patterns of conditioned responses to their environment. This is a function of the first or lower signal system. Having accomplished that as, for example, when the soldier is taught how to behave under certain circumstances during training, individuals develop within the second or higher signal system a set of triggers or signals based on words, signs, feelings, or other designators that are quite separate from the physical stimuli that created the original patterns of response. By properly utilizing the second signal system, people can trigger the original response patterns. Lest one not take any of this seriously, it should be noted that the Russian word for "education" is the same as the word for "training." According to the Soviets, education does not mean the ability to explore one's intellectual abilities free of restraint as much as it implies the need to shape or mold the thinking processes to produce correct thought and behavior. The Soviet system of education and military psychology is based on the same premises, that individuals or soldiers can be taught or "oriented" to certain behaviors that are then reinforced in the brain by a second set of signals. When these second signals are triggered, the original response results.

The same principles apply in the training of the soldier. The initial stimuli of his training experience act on a body receptor and travel to the brain into the cerebral cortex. It is here that a "zone of excitement" is created and radiation or induction occurs. Under this condition the cerebral cortex spreads or diffuses the original excitation of the nerve fibers into neighboring areas of the brain, "thereby bringing the nervous system to a state of high activity."[8] The process of radiation can result in further excitement or inhibition, and it is here that the location of the will is found which properly controls and channels excitement or inhibition. When nervous activity is heightened, a condition of positive induction occurs. When nervous activity in the brain is reduced, negative induction occurs. The reaction of the individual to a given stimulus, either to heighten or depress activity, is a consequence of the pattern of previous conditioning to which he or she has been exposed, disciplined by the will. Changes in mood and psychic orientation result from disturbances in the balance between excitation and inhibition as biological processes of the cerebral cortex. Any excitation of the brain causes psychic tension, namely, stress or anxiety. If the will fails and excitation becomes too extreme, there is too much radiation into other centers of the brain, and extreme conditions, such as fear, may result. If too little radiation occurs, then depression results. The point is that the whole process of nervous radiation, either hyper-excitement or hyper-depression, is rooted in the cerebral cortex of the brain, and the entire process is physiological without any unconscious or subconscious factors involved.

Critical to the soldier's ability to control his mental activity under battle conditions is the concept of will or, what the Soviets term, volitional strength. Will is "the apex of the human psyche" and consists in a person's ability to control his or her actions in accordance with learned convictions, goals, and moral and political principles. Will is the basis of all correct social conduct and human activity. In the formation of the will, Soviet military psychiatrists maintain that the most important factor is the soldier's recognition and understanding of the higher socially significant goals for which he acts, a point to which we will return later. Soviet psychiatrists talk of individuals who have weak or "evil" wills. A weak will develops when the individual does not understand correct duties or socially significant goals. The soldier who is improperly conditioned to social norms and duties suffers from a weak will. On the battlefield, a soldier who lacks a strong will risks having his "organic needs" take over and direct his behavior, as, for example, the organism's need to survive. Under conditions of great stress, the organism may flee or otherwise break down as a way of ensuring its survival, rather than having the strength of will to stand and fight in the service of larger and more significant goals and duties.

The will is a socially acquired conditioned reflex located in the cerebral cortex. It is a function of the second signal system which governs all volitional activities. The first reflex is located in the primary signal system and is directly connected to the original stimulus. The secondary signal stimuli—words, speech, thoughts, signs, and so on—are developed in the secondary signal system which triggers the original pattern of trained response, although the original stimuli may be absent. Thus, the soldier is exposed and conditioned to respond to live fire. But after this exposure, repeated several times, it is his second signal system which further governs his behavior. The command "Don't run under fire" is an instruction that tells the brain what to do when the organism is exposed to fire. The self-generated command is a function of the second signal system.

Soldiers are conditioned to certain kinds of behavior by exposing them to circumstances they understand—the orienting response—

which lays the groundwork for establishing the original patterns of conditioned response. The soldier's initial exposure to extreme events is called the "dynamic stereotype," a term defining the most prominent stimuli to which the soldier must learn to adapt. If the soldier encounters conditions for which he is untrained or cannot foresee (improper orienting), a high degree of psychic tension results which, if left unresolved, can lead to strong negative reactions and battle psychosis.

In Soviet military psychology, the soldier's temperament is an important background variable against which other variables interact. The importance of temperament, defined as a mental state, is that certain psychiatric types ought not to be placed in some situations without running the risk of extreme mental aberration. The concept of temperament is important to Soviet military psychological thought and is defined as "the property of personality which expresses the dynamic features of its mental activity."[9] It is one of the basic characteristics of an individual's system of nervous activity and influences the other operations of the personality and mental processes.

It should be stressed again here that the personality of the soldier, as with all his other mental functions, is based on the physiology of the brain. Temperament is perceived as a physiologically based property that depends on "the particular features of higher nervous activity; the basic nervous process that is innervation and excitation and upon their relationship."[10] In short, temperament is a key element of the personality which helps determine the soldier's ability to respond to certain extreme conditions. It is dependent on three basic elements: (1) the strength of the nervous system to tolerate stress without disrupting the nervous activity of the brain; (2) the equilibrium of the nervous process to adequately balance excitation and inhibition, thus preventing extremes of mental activity; and (3) the mobility of the nervous process to quickly disperse stimulation and organize the conditioned reflex to adjust to changing environments.[11] On this basis, the Soviets identify four basic types of personality temperament: the sanguine, choleric, phlegmatic, and melancholic.

The importance of temperament as a concept in Soviet psychological thought is its ability to provide a major background variable against which psychiatrists can deal with disruptions of the nervous processes associated with mental activity. The Soviets are clearly aware that individuals have different personality characteristics that endow them with different behavioral abilities. They also acknowledge that some of these characteristics are formed very early in life and that others result from defective conditioning. They also acknowledge that, in some cases, these personality traits are very difficult, if not impossible, to reverse with additional counterconditioning.

Soviet military psychologists and psychophysiologists will admit that certain personality types are more fit for some activities than for others. As noted earlier, a certain amount of psychological testing is aimed at determining what types of individuals are best suited for certain tasks, although such testing is confined to a small number of highly skilled tasks, say astronauts and pilots. There is no evidence of any widespread testing among the military population in general. They also understand that personality traits set practical, if not theoretical, limits on the conditioning process and the way in which certain types will respond to extreme environmental changes even after they have been conditioned. But, in a practical sense, none of this has too much impact on the practice of military psychiatry in the Soviet Union. Personality traits or not, the soldier is still held rigidly responsible for all his actions.

EMOTIONS

The Soviets view emotions as physiological reactions of the organism to external stimuli. Emotions are perceived as reflections of objective reality and are termed "reflections in a man's brain to very real experiences."[12] Soviet psychiatrists acknowledge that emotions are among the strongest excitations of the brain and that they tend to manifest themselves in a number of external behavioral signs, including timbre of the voice, paralysis, and panic. Objective reality is what is at the base of emotions, and they are essentially very strong excitations of the cerebral cortex provoked by stimuli of the second signal system. But the Soviets emphasize that individuals can control their emotions by disciplining their second signal system through the volition of will. Emotions help mobilize what the Soviets call "spiritual or moral forces" that help attain socially significant goals or spur social activity. They also recognize that the power of emotions can be negative in that they can hinder proper conduct. In Soviet psychiatric thought, emotions are seen to be governed by the same objective laws of stimulus-response conditioning that govern all other types of human behavior. Emotions change the physiological state of the nervous system, and this change can be disciplined and directed to resist certain kinds of stimuli and be more accommodating to others.

As with all other physiological reactions, emotions are aimed at achieving goals. Once the nervous system is excited, that is, put in an emotional state, the brain searches the environment for evidence that it has achieved or is at least nearing the achievement of the goal for which the stimulus originally activated the nervous system. If evidence arrives fairly quickly that it is achieving its goal, need satisfaction results and a positive emotional state is generated. If habitual patterns of activity are disturbed and there is a long delay in need satisfaction, nervous tension intensifies in the center of the brain and negative emotion is produced. This condition sets the stage for emotional exhaustion. A normal person can sustain a state of excited nervous emotional activity for only a short period of time after which either calm or depression will set in. The reason for this is that the "energy" of stimulated nerve signals gradually depletes itself as a result of chemical activity, and the nerve cells shift into a depressive state. If negative emotion persists, extremes of emotion occur, and a soldier can become incapable of moving at all or made to panic. The point is that the emotional process is not subjective but objective in the sense that it is a physiologically based, patterned conditioned response to external stimuli outside the brain. It is transmitted by physiological means and can be controlled by a disciplined will located in the second signal system.

Emotions are subjective only in the sense that the physiology that makes up the organic functions of the brain and the personality is either properly or improperly trained to sustain different degrees of nervous excitement. This is very much the key to understanding the training of the will given to each Soviet soldier, a subject that is discussed later in this book. Given the assumption that the brain is subject to conditioned response, the soldier must be trained to acquire certain patterned responses to deal with the extreme conditions of battle which otherwise could excite his emotions too much or depress them to the point of paralysis.

Military psychologists identify three general emotional states: moods, affects, and passions.[13] Moods are defined as generally weak expressions of positive or negative feelings that last a relatively long time, perhaps for days or even weeks. Such moods can range from a general feeling of well-being to a feeling of malaise. Moods seem to constitute a general emotional condition and serve as a background against which other more intense behaviors and emotions can occur. Passions, on the other hand, are seen as strong emotional forces that are always goal directed. In the training doctrine of the Soviet military, two central goals are emphasized: the soldier's love of the motherland and his hatred of the enemy. The military tries very hard to instill these two goals as objects of passionate emotions by continual propaganda and political meetings, so that the soldier knows—is "oriented" in a Pavlovian sense—to the goals for which he fights. The most important of the three emotional states are affective states. An affective state is defined as a highly charged emotional state characterized by a gradual increase in the intensity of the stimuli in an almost unrestrained manner that leads to a clear external behavioral expression.

Affects are experiences of great force, but of brief duration, and are characterized by changes in consciousness and a disruption of volitional control. Note that the Soviets define an affective state *ab initio* as one in which volitional control is challenged and consciousness is clouded. Examples of affective states are extreme anger, terror, and fear. Such states are characterized by strong stimuli to which a person cannot readily adapt as a consequence of improper training or conditioning. Control of affective states can be achieved by a strongly developed will which can either distract or change the individual's attention by "transferring a portion of strong nervous excitation to other areas of the brain."[14] Soviet theory holds that an extremely strong excitation of the cerebral cortex can disrupt the personality if it radiates out from the cortical control centers and creates conditions of great tension within other areas of the brain. Eventually, such a situation leads to emotional collapse.

Psychiatrists define two types of emotions (as distinguished from emotional states): sthenic and asthenic. A sthenic emotion is a pure physiological stimulation that activates increased levels of nervous physiological activity. It is, in short, a severe physiological shock to the brain that completely disrupts its ability to function properly.

Asthenic emotions are characterized by abnormal decreases in the ability of the nerve cells of the cerebral cortex to transmit excitation. Whereas sthenic emotions lead to hyper-excitability, asthenic emotions lead to a depressed state, such as melancholia. Panic, for example, is based on the sthenic emotions, whereas fear or torpor is based on the asthenic emotions.

The Soviets stress that emotions are tied to activity within the second signal system. They call these cortical emotions, which they distinguish from subcortical emotions which are rooted in pure physiological reactions to external stimuli. The distinguishing characteristic of cortical emotions is precisely their consciousness in the sense that the individual experiencing the emotion realizes what is happening to him. If, as in the case of the soldier, he is assumed to be aware of the development and onset of emotional states, then there is both rationality and accountability for his actions. Because cortical emotions are tied to the rational operations of the second signal system, "the reasons which cause them are always clear to man and can be expressed in words."[15] Consequently, the soldier is perceived to be aware of the development of extreme emotional states that might lead to breakdown or panic. He is thus responsible for his actions. This concept squares well with the Marxist notion of the individual as rational and having control over his or her actions at all times.

Cortical emotions are also called higher emotions. Chief among them, in the Soviet view, as they affect the conditioning of the soldier are the moral feelings that are rooted in social historical goals, the development of the soldier's personality, and an awareness of the larger historical context of Marxist-Leninism. The Soviets maintain that soldiers who have proper ideological motivation, that is, who have correctly perceived and oriented themselves to the knowledge of higher social goals, are expected to use this knowledge as the basis for developing adequate volitional strength to control their emotions. Although this may appear bizarre to Western military psychiatrists, their Soviet counterparts hold this view very seriously, and it is a premise strongly based in Marxist thought. The idea is that soldiers are rational in that they are goal oriented. They are, therefore, not irrational in the sense of being moved by their subconscious or unconscious as in Freudian psychiatry. The Soviet military, therefore, spends a great deal of time indoctrinating their soldiers as to their "higher socially significant goals." Without an awareness of these goals, the soldier cannot be expected to develop reasonably adequate patterns of conditioned behavior that develop the will, which can then control and mitigate the potentially disruptive effects of strong emotional excitation.

For the Soviets, education is a process of mental molding and attitude formation rather than free exploration. Hence, they pay close attention—not only politically, but also sociologically and psychologically—to developing the soldier's conscious awareness of why he must fight and sacrifice. Without the presence of these goals, rational action is impossible, and if rational action is impossible, then so, too, is the development of a strong will. Under these conditions, no soldier can be expected to withstand the horrors of battle. Marxist theory, military psychiatry, and the training programs of the Soviet soldier are all of one piece.

This "rational" approach to emotional shock implies that the soldier is always responsible for his actions, even under conditions of great emotional stress. Soviet military psychiatry defines military shock as "a stormy emotional experience accompanied by disorderly conduct."[16] Military psychiatrists believe that shock is an extremely powerful force but that it is generally temporary in that its "manifestations cannot long persist and quickly outlives itself."[17] Shock is temporary because the overstimulation of the central nervous system quickly exhausts the energy of the nerve cells which reduces their ability to transmit impulses. The stronger the shock, the greater the slowdown which follows it, leading to exhaustion and fatigue. Exhaustion as a consequence of emotional shock is accompanied by a "partial narrowing of consciousness and a loss of control over action and deed accomplishment."[18] However, it is important to emphasize again the rational aspects of Soviet military psychiatry because this narrowing of consciousness does not in any way diminish the soldier's responsibility for his actions.

The Soviets point out that "affect never advances unexpectedly but moves in stages" which a well-trained soldier should be able to recognize and, through his will buttressed by volitional training, be able to control. "Most often man allows himself to enter into an affective state and therefore he is responsible for everything that happens in that affective state."[19] This is important. Although military psychiatrists recognize battleshock as a phenomenon, they see it resulting from improper training, a character defect in the soldier, or the soldier's unwillingness or inability to develop proper volitional strength. Paradoxically, although the Soviets are determinists in a larger sense, they insist that the responsibility for one's actions remains even under conditions of battleshock. This goes a long way in explaining why the Soviet treatment of battleshock is so much more severe than in the West. Whether or not the soldier remembers what he has done, he remains responsible to his superiors for his actions. In a functional sense, this is equivalent to defining soldiers suffering from battleshock as cowards or shirkers and dealing with them accordingly. This definition is based not on an arbitrary social definition of cowardice, but on a theory of the psychological and psychiatric operations of the human personality. In that sense, it goes quite beyond what some allied armies did in World War I when they used social definitions of cowardice in order to deal with the problem of battleshock. The Western definition was socially derived with little empirical basis. The Soviet definition is a clinical definition anchored in psychiatric theory.

FEAR, PANIC, COWARDICE, AND HEROISM

As noted earlier, the way in which military psychiatrists expect soldiers to behave will determine the diagnostic criteria used in the field. In turn, the diagnostic criteria will determine the methodologies of treatment. It is interesting to examine the way Soviet psychiatric theorists see the phenomena of fear, panic, cowardice, and heroism because nowhere else does one so clearly encounter the strong physiological and organic predispositions of military psychiatrists to define human behavior in such stark physical terms. For example, the Soviets regard fear as a strong emotional state caused by extremely strong stimuli often posing a threat to the organism. Fear often manifests itself as acute motor excitation accompanied by an exaggerated desire to flee. Another form of fear may cause a soldier to become rigid and be completely incapable of movement. This hyper-fear or terror causes disorientation and profound physiological disturbances in the brain. Fear is the result of extreme tension in the brain of the soldier, resulting largely from his having to adjust to unanticipated circumstances. This tension becomes so acute that it disorders the mental processes. This disordering is a consequence of an improperly trained and conditioned second signal system which is incapable of controlling severe and rapid nervous radiation in the brain.

The nature of cowardly action is expressed in similar terms. Under great stress, the emotions reach a state of great excitement and bypass the cortex where the second signal system can regulate the nervous activity by inhibition. With no inhibitory action to stop the nervous excitement by imposing on it volitional restraining action, a direct motor response may set in and the individual soldier may flee or go rigid. Soviet military psychiatrists draw heavily on Pavlov in basing fear and cowardice in the physiology of the brain and agree with Pavlov that "that which is psychologically called fear, cowardice, and timidity has its own physiological substratum in the inhibitive state in the larger hemispheres which represent various degrees of the passive defensive reflex."[20] Cowardice has nothing to do with character in the way the term is used in the West. It has to do with deranged physiology.

Soviet military psychiatrists, of course, reject "bourgeois theories" about the psychological causes of fear and panic. They reject the notion, for example, that fear and panic are caused by either the manifestation of an instinct for self-preservation (the biological or instinctual explanation), or the impact of contagion on the group (the sociological explanation). They reject the view that panic and fear result from anything except objective conditions linked to organic disruptions of the thought and volitional processes. Thus, "the cause of panic is not blind imitation but above all a decline in a level of motivation and the dulling of self-control."[21] Such events as fear and panic occur when physiological reactions become so strong that they destroy emotional stability by disrupting the mental processes in the cerebral cortex. The soldier who runs or breaks under fire is one whose second signal system has been improperly conditioned. There is no validity accorded the view that fear and panic are normal reactions of normal human beings under great stress.

Soviet military psychiatrists distinguish between certain lower biological acts, such as fright, and those acts such as fear, panic, and shock which are centered in the second signal system. They suggest that fright is an unconditioned reflex reaction that occurs when a stimulus is so overpowering that it generalizes itself in the brain and triggers the body automatically into a "defense function contributing to the mobilization of all the resources of the organism"[22] in order to escape from the stimulus. Fright or frightful shock is not a conscious act, but the action of the body acting autogenically so that the organism flees in order to avoid being destroyed. This notion of autogenic action is stood on its head in Soviet military training where it is held that when the soldier is properly conditioned he may, under conditions of great stress, continue to operate automatically, and even unconsciously, in carrying out his military duties.

When fear reaches the level of hyper-fear, the soldier goes into psychological shock, a profound and pathological form of fear defined as the "temporary loss of any ability for mental activity in persons who are psychologically unprepared for modern war."[23] (Note the emphasis on improper training.) Consciousness narrows as stress increases until it becomes impossible for a soldier to carry out his duties. Nonetheless, the Soviets accept the proposition that some stress may be useful; they believe that "psychic tension" (stress) is very helpful to the soldier. Psychic tension is defined as a condition in which a stimulus impacts on the physiology of the nervous system and the brain to bring the brain to moderate level of excitement. For every activity there is an optimal emotional tension level that allows performance at the highest level of efficiency. In this view, stress is an omnipresent biological characteristic of all human action in the sense that it implies the excitation of the cerebral cortex which is required for all conscious behavior. The only question is how well one controls stress.

Similarly, panic arises in the second signal system and is also a volitional act. The Soviets maintain that panic arises largely from the soldier's lack of information about the threat he is facing. This leads to an inaccurate and exaggerated notion of the danger he must confront. In Pavlovian terms, the organism is not properly oriented to its environment in that it does not discern those stimuli with which it must deal. In addition, panic is seen as a social phenomenon in terms of contagion, and is not caused by a group instinct. Contagion or panic results only when men in a group suffer from the same inaccurate and exaggerated information and, when together, their minds perceive conditions that are not present. Contagion is the result of a group suffering from an improper orienting reflex.

Not unexpectedly, fear and panic are seen as defects in the soldier's character resulting from improper conditioning and training. This produces a physiological defect in the improperly conditioned nerve pathways in the second signal system of the cerebral cortex. The corollary of this position is that one can condition men to deal with fear and panic by proper training. Furthermore, a direct responsibility is placed on the well-trained soldier to control his fear. The more experience a soldier has, the less fearful he is expected to be and the less likely he is to break under stress. This particular proposition of Soviet psychiatry, while logically deducible from the propositions dealing with the physiological basis of fear and panic, is probably doubtful. It certainly flies in the face of research published by David Marlowe and others which suggests that, whereas there are significant differences in the rates of psychiatric breakdown between inexperienced soldiers and seasoned veterans, over time the differences disappear.[24] Nonetheless, in both training doctrine and psychiatric theory, the Soviets maintain that fear and panic can be eliminated entirely by proper ideological and "moral combat training."

Soviet psychiatrists have identified some of the causes of battlefield stress. They are much the same as those cited in Western psychiatric thought and include: (1) danger that creates a threat to life, (2) the responsibility for carrying out one's mission, (3) ambiguity in the information surrounding the organism, (4) insufficient time for making decisions, (5) excessive emotional excitability as a consequence of defective character or training, (6) placement of a soldier in a situation for which he has not been properly trained or conditioned, (7) a soldier's lack of confidence in his weapons, and (8) a degree of isolation from the collective.[25] Western military psychiatrists agree that all of these factors precipitate battle stress. The difference is that, for the Soviets, the impact of these factors on the organism will depend on the ability of the cerebral cortex to deal with excessive stimulation. In short, the crucial variable is the physiology of the brain rather than the soldier's subjective emotional response.

In light of the research conducted by Reuven Gal of the Israeli Defense Force and others on heroism and its causes, it is interesting to ask how the Soviets explain heroic action under fire.[26] It will be recalled that Soviet psychiatric theory rejects the usual motivations that have been used to explain heroism in the West. For instance, they reject as bourgeois the idea that group cohesion and the bonds among men in the group are capable of forming in the absence of a higher ideological awareness. As such, one cannot use such elements as love and respect of peers to explain heroism in Soviet units. In addition, they reject the Freudian notion of unconscious and personal motivations such as self-interest, prestige, the desire to be loved and respected by others, and even the desire to die or commit suicide. The Soviets cannot explain heroism by hidden motivations. Furthermore, the Soviet military psychiatrists also reject the prospect that a soldier might go beserk or react almost instinctively or unconsciously in performing an act of heroism. What, then, are the causes of heroism?

Heroism is seen as residing in the conscious and rationally developed "achievement of a designated goal of particularly important societal significance."[27] Soviet soldiers are expected to be motivated by those higher social goals that are seen as crucial to disciplining the second signal system. It is in the second signal system that the highest forms of emotional and rational attachments to higher goals are formed. Accordingly, in the Soviet view, heroism proceeds from rational action by the soldier which is the product of one of two basic higher goals: (1) an intense love of the motherland or (2) a deep hatred of the enemy. Soviet military psychiatry offers no concept of the soldier acting, as S.L.A. Marshall suggests, out of love or respect for one's peers or even out of unconscious motives in performing heroic acts. Heroism is seen as a patently rational act to which men are capable of being trained. It is an act of conscious self-abnegation as an extension of the soldier's ideological commitment. Thus, "readiness of heroic feats at the cost of one's own blood and even one's own life is the most vivid manifestation of ideological conviction, honor and nobility in a man."[28]

Clearly, Soviet psychiatric theory on fear, panic, cowardice, and heroism is fundamentally different from Western theory. Among Western military psychiatrists, these states can usually be expected to occur at a given statistical level within any unit under certain levels of stress. None of these phenomena is completely preventable, being likely to manifest themselves regardless of any measure taken. Although it is possible within limits—and these limits have yet to be fully explored—to train a soldier to handle certain levels of stress, by and large whatever objective conditions of stress the soldier must face must first be filtered and interpreted by those subjective psychological dispositions that comprise the soldier's personality. The same stressful situations are likely to have differential impacts on different soldiers. Furthermore, in the Soviet view, American psychiatrists tend to be biased in their views by their deep personality explanations for human behavior. By contrast, the Soviets see behavior on the battlefield as resulting from proper conditioning which develops the second signal system and makes it possible for the organism to resist stress at high levels. It is all very straightforward and "scientific."

Although Western armies have made some detailed studies on the prevention of stress casualties, the Soviets have made greater efforts to develop a rather complete set of axioms on the subject. These axioms are firmly embedded in their training doctrine, if less so in practice. Because the Soviets assume that the individual is infinitely malleable and that human actions are always rational and conscious, Soviet military psychiatrists have understandably given more attention to the problem of preventing stress breakdown.

5
Preventing Battle Stress

The Soviets are acutely aware of the potential stress of modern warfare, even conventional wars. The stress levels and accompanying breakdown rates would, of course, be worse in the event of nuclear warfare. Until 1967, the Soviets gave little attention to battle stress, and their tactical doctrine affirmed that large-scale conventional military operations within a nuclear context could not realistically be conducted. Until that time, the political and military leadership had maintained that any war fought between the superpowers would be nuclear and that conventional forces would play only a minor and secondary role.

Between 1967 and 1972, the Soviets radically modified their tactical doctrine and their strategic view of massive retaliation, returning to their earlier experiences from World War II. Soviet doctrine now assets that, even in a nuclear war, large-scale conventional military operations are possible and will actually be decisive once the initial exchange of nuclear weapons has occurred. Hence, after 1967 the Soviet military began to think very seriously about the problem of dealing with the high levels of battle stress casualties that would accompany modern war. This change in emphasis led the Soviet military establishment to provide financial and political support to a number of new initiatives designed to reestablish military psychology.

The Soviets have given a great deal of thought to preventing breakdown among soldiers in battle by immunizing them against stress. They have also expanded their theoretical doctrine on protecting military forces against stress. As already noted, this doctrine derives from Marxist theory and from a physiological perception of the human personality and psyche. The Soviets' approach has taken four basic directions. (1) They make use of social conditioning, which is seen to result from the soldier's total life history, namely, the creation of a new "socialist man" with a changed human nature motivated by appropriate social and historic attitudes and goals. (2) Soldiers are exposed to very realistic battle training in order to "orient the organism" to the horrors of the battlefield. Drawing heavily on Pavlov, the Soviets maintain that no soldier can be expected to perform well under fire if he encounters conditions for which he is not trained. In Pavlovian terms, the soldier must be oriented to the realities he will encounter if he is to adequately cope with them. (3) Relatively simple battle engagement doctrines and training in rote battle drills have been developed so as to routinize the tasks the soldier will have to perform under stress. (4) Since 1972, Soviet military psychiatrists have begun serious explorations of drug use in order to find a chemical solution to maintaining the manpower strength of their fighting units. They have used both psychostimulators to increase performance and tranquilizers to treat and reduce battleshock. Some drugs are also used as prophylactics to prevent the initial onset of stress. The ultimate goal of the Soviet program to combat battle stress is to conserve manpower by preventing the breakdown of soldiers in the first place and treating and returning soldiers to the battle as quickly as possible. Overlaying the entire program is the Soviet use of harsh battlefield discipline in order to reinforce the soldier's conditioning and training.

The Soviets' immunizing conditioning program has targeted four emotional or mental states in the soldier: surprise, fear, fatigue, and pain. The Soviet system of conditioning, training, and discipline attempts to deal with these states by developing a number of conditioned reflexes within the soldier in order to help him cope with the disruption of his mental processes.

In Soviet military psychiatric theory, teaching the soldier to deal with surprise means exposing him to and informing him about the horrors of war he can expect to confront. It requires training him as realistically as possible so that he knows what to expect from his own and his enemy's weapons. The attempt to create a conditioned mental state is based heavily on the physiological concept developed by Pavlov and others than an organism can only adapt to its environment when its orientation reflex is properly prepared, that is, when the soldier understands what will happen under fire and is trained to react to these conditions. The ability to cope is a reflex acquired through training and conditioning. Therefore, the Soviets try to prevent and reduce the mental state of surprise by harsh and realistic training and by informing the soldier of the true nature of battle as realistically as possible. Indeed, modern Soviet doctrine in this regard derives very much from the old training doctrine developed by the generals of Catherine the Great. Their training doctrine was summed up in the motto "Difficult in peace, easy in war."

The other mental states—fear, fatigue, and pain—are elements which one would normally expect in a conditioning program. Fear, as has been stated, belongs to the second signal system and is distinguished from flight, which is a reflex located in the lower biological reflex system. Panic is also a second signal system response for which the soldier is always held responsible. Fear results not from any objective reality, but from subjective interpretations of that reality. Accordingly, the soldier is conditioned against fear by "knowing" what will happen to him under fire. Soviet military psychiatrists see fear as a gradual process wherein the soldier is consciously aware of what is happening to him and still allows this emotional state to overwhelm him. Consequently, Soviet doctrine holds the soldier responsible for recognizing the onset of fear and stopping it. Unlike flight, panic and fear are not rooted in the lower reflexes but in the conditioned trained reflexes of the second signal system. Thus, they are conscious states for which the soldier is rationally responsible in dealing with their consequences.

Fatigue also affects the soldier's ability to function well. Lack of sleep and overwork lessen the soldier's ability to process information and to make decisions, which, in turn, leads to confusion and a deterioration of the soldier's volitional strength (will). The Soviets try to condition their soldiers to cope by building into their tactical doctrine mandatory sleep and rest periods before an attack. A close examination of Soviet battle performance during World War II demonstrates the inaccuracy of the commonly held Western notion of Soviet forces as a steamroller marching continuously against the German Army. Soviet tactics were marked by a series of combat pulses occurring after long periods of prolonged buildup and rest. Soviet units, usually of army or corps size, would customarily build up their strength and rest their men during relatively long periods and then conduct the attack in a highly intense manner until clearly defined objectives were attained. Soviet units would then often stop and rest again, even though, at times, a continuation of the attack would have been able to gain further advances. This practice accounts for the perceptions of German officers that Soviet units almost always failed to exploit their advances. It is much more correct to describe the successful Soviet performance in World War II as a series of intense hammer blows than as a continuous steamroller. Soviet military psychiatrists see mandatory rest periods as crucial to reducing the effects of fatigue. When coupled with excellent physical fitness developed through the DOSAAF system and good selection prior to entering military service, the Soviet practice of enforcing mandatory rest and sleep periods is likely to go a long way in reducing fatigue.

Soviet military psychiatrists always consider pain within the context of battlefield operations in that the soldier is expected to endure very arduous battle conditions and great physical discomfort. Endurance of physical pain is stressed. In a broader context, however, the Soviets try to condition their soldiers to the fact that military life is hard and battle even worse. Discomfort and pain are seen as normal and integral parts of sustained battlefield operations. In training, the Soviet soldier is exposed to very severe conditions so that when he encounters them on the field of battle, they are no stranger to him.

Armies of the West do very little training in stress prevention. In general, the West "conducts" this training through unit cohesion, officer leadership, and horizontal bonding. By contrast, the Soviets have developed a well-integrated theory of stress, detailing how it acts on the soldier and the specific reflexes that must be developed in order to prevent and control its debilitating effects. Soviet combat psychiatrists have delineated what the soldier should and should not do under stressful situations. As Christopher Donnelly notes,

Preventing Battle Stress

It is the effective stress on the individual soldier and, through him, on the Soviet military system that modern Soviet military doctrine takes so much into account. There is no single feature of the Soviet attitude toward stress of battle and its effect on man and the military machine that could really be called revolutionary or even that is unique to the Soviet Army. What makes for a special Soviet approach is a combination of attitudes, the recognition of the problem and a conscious effort to deal with it.[1]

In this regard, it must be said that Soviet military training and combat psychiatry are much more closely intertwined in terms of theory and practice than seems to be the case in most armies of the West, with the possible exception of the Israeli Army.

SOCIAL CONDITIONING

The Soviet soldier receives a great deal of social conditioning even before he enters military service; this conditioning is a major factor in military training. The larger social conditioning of the citizen is regarded as an integral part of training their soldiers to withstand the rigors of battle. This mechanism is taken very seriously and, indeed, may even be the most seriously regarded way to train the soldier to withstand stress.

Notions of psychological conditioning for military service in the West and Soviet Union are radically different. In the West, psychological conditioning for military service is generally obtained only in the military itself and not in civilian life. Whatever training is acquired during military service is expected to last only as long as one remains in the military, and it is expected to deteriorate once the soldier is released. To the extent that military training in the West is conditioning at all, it is aimed at rather specific conditions found only in the military and relates to those conditions encountered on the battlefield. Western societies have no systematic psychological conditioning programs for military service. More importantly, in the West the acquired military mind set is expected to be exercised only within the military context and, when one leaves it, it is seen as somewhat useless.

In the USSR, as already suggested, psychological conditioning for military service is seen as a continuation of the larger social conditioning received in civilian life. The entire process of preparing a man for battle is seen as cumulative and continuous beginning in civilian life, extended in the military, and continuing when the soldier leaves military service. This is precisely what is meant by the Soviet concept of a "nation in arms." The basis is the same, namely, proper behavior in any context is based on objective reality as interpreted by the doctrine of Marx and Lenin. The central feature of psychological motivation, whether civilian or military, is the "high ideological and theoretical preparedness" of the soldier or the citizen. Accordingly, "in the psychological structure of an individual soldier or collective the motives for their conduct are decisive, that is the social values, convictions, ideals as well as high moral political patriotic internationalist feelings and party political work. The entire system of ideological political indoctrination and the moral political preparation of military personnel play the main role in forming these motives."[2] In short, the formula is "man-collective-military machine" with each level seen as being built on the rest. The Soviets do not believe that the soldier can, in a meaningful way, be separated from the social and political structure and the life he lives in the larger society. The idea of military performance as rooted in the experiences and attachments of men within their military units apart from any larger social and political motives and values is rejected as bourgeois doctrine and as incorrect.

Whereas in the West the soldier's ability to withstand stress is seen as a characteristic of the whole personality, in the USSR this ability is expressed more in terms of the soldier's ability to carry out specific tasks under stress which vary from soldier to soldier and service to service. Where the Western view involves personality formation or character as a general condition, the Soviet view requires the inculcation of military skills within the larger context of social conditioning.

Professor Donnelly notes that the West often underestimates the effect of ideological conditioning on the Soviet soldier.[3] Like any religious belief, Communist ideology and values provide a broad moral basis or general perspective through which many other things are judged. It must also be noted that there are really no alternatives to the official view of the world in a totalitarian society, and it is this official view to which the child and adult are constantly exposed. Nor are there any effective ways to develop alternative world outlooks. Furthermore, the concept of a "nation in arms" is a basic tenet of Marxist-Leninism wherein the whole population is expected to defend the revolution and the state in order to defeat any aggression. This concept does not mean only maintaining a large military force. It requires the militarization of the whole society and the development of a war-making capacity in order to defend the revolution from the attacks of capitalist countries.

The complete centralized control of the Communist Party with its cadre critically positioned in every sector of Soviet society provides an opportunity for coordinated integration of all elements of society, which is simply impossible in the West. This control facilitates the effective militarization of the society and its economy. The readiness of the Soviet population to accept the militarization of their economy and social life can be achieved only by maintaining a high level of military awareness among the population itself. The society is militarized to an extent which Westerners often find difficult to believe. This is most evident in the training and indoctrination of Soviet youth.

Soviet youth are far more isolated from their foreign contemporaries than youth in any Western country. Visitors to the Soviet Union are often shocked to discover that Soviet citizens routinely accept the regime's often biased and sometimes bizarre official explanations offered about events in the West. There are no other ways of determining what reality is except through the regime's official pronouncements.

From his earliest days, the Soviet child is taught about the glory of Soviet military exploits and victories. Upon entering school, he is exposed regularly to military and patriotic themes. He is expected to become a member of the Octobrists, an organization made up of children under nine years of age who wear pins bearing the likeness of Lenin as a young man and who are taught that their goal in life is to defend the Soviet Revolution. Once youths reach the ages of ten to fourteen years, about 90 percent of them become members of the junior party organization called the Pioneers, a highly militarized organization that provides an annual summer camp where children are exposed to rudimentary military training. The summer camp program is called Zaranitza, which means "battle lightning." In these summer sessions, Soviet children are taught the rudiments of military tactics and exercises, and are exposed to military men who direct their activities. By the age of seventeen, the Soviet youth is likely to become a member of the Komsomol, the senior party youth organization whose important task it is to prepare youth for military service through its close ties with the DOSAAF system of premilitary training.

The DOSAAF program requires young men to undergo 140 hours of basic military training while at school and work. Females also take part in this training. In addition, all Soviet children are exposed to civil defense training. Probably 75 percent of the older age cohort receive effective military training at this point. Even the physical training in civilian schools has a decided military tenor. This training is called BGTO, which translates as "be ready for labor and defense." To attain a certificate of proficiency as a Komsomol member at the age of sixteen, young men and women must pass the BGTO test. The military theme of the test is reflected in the requirement that young people be proficient at throwing a hand grenade 25 meters.[4] All of the youths' training is designed to inculcate in them a sense of military duty, and the training is constantly reinforced by political indoctrination and the overall integration of the military and civilian elements in all walks of life.

In addition to early military training, Soviet youth are involved in a widespread civil defense organization that serves as a further mechanism for integrating civilian and military life. Military commanders of local garrisons automatically hold office in the local administrative and decision-making councils of government in which the garrisons are located. Furthermore, Soviet youth are taught that military industry takes priority over civilian concerns in economic life. In addition, the military medical service constitutes the senior branch of the Soviet national health system, and all aspects of the public health system are closely integrated to support military needs. Taken together, military life is seen as a kind of capstone to the life of the Soviet youth, one that builds on the prior conditioning in supporting state goals they received as children. Moreover, military life is viewed as a basic integrative mechanism for bringing all aspects of social conditioning together toward the goal of defending the revolution and the state against its enemies. It is all part of the Soviet view that a new socialist man with a different human nature can be created, a man who is committed to the defense of his homeland, one who truly hates the enemy and, perhaps most important, one who is willing to endure great hardships and even sacrifice his life to preserve Communist ideals. Some idea of both the extremity and thoroughness of Soviet societal conditioning can be gained from noting that a new bride is expected to place her bridal bouquet at the site of the local war memorial as an expression of her support for the goals of the Soviet state. Finally, it must be understood as well that absolutely no antimilitary sentiment is either appreciated or tolerated in the Soviet Union.

Taken together, the average Soviet citizen from his youngest days until he is ready to enter military service is exposed to a great deal of background conditioning designed to inculcate in him those values and ideals which the Soviet regime defines as "higher social motives." The Soviets clearly reject the view that one can be both a good soldier and a bad citizen. Performance as a soldier is seen as an extension of the values and sentiments developed as a citizen. In military service one is expected to be motivated by the same set of values that motivates the civilian and vice versa. When it is recalled that a major premise of Soviet psychiatry is that man is rational and that rationality means the ability to act on the basis of one's internalized and consciously realized social-historic goals, then however odd the Soviet notion of social conditioning may appear to the Western mind, within the Soviet context it is a perfectly logical system.

Assessing the effectiveness of the social conditioning of the Soviet soldier is difficult for several reasons. First, data on the attitudes of the Soviet soldiers toward political conditioning are scarce. In all the years in which military analysts and academics have been studying the Soviet Union, only the three works by this author offer any data based on actual interviews with Soviet soldiers themselves, that even remotely touch this question. Second, any data on this question occurs in a vacuum, that is, quite apart from circumstances where the Soviet Union is at war. As in most countries, love of one's homeland and patriotism are far more in evidence when a country is under siege than in peacetime.

These difficulties notwithstanding, we should take note of the findings of *The Mind of the Soviet Fighting Man*, available as of this writing, which relate the question of ideological conditioning directly to Soviet soldiers. The data must be approached with caution, but when taken together they suggest that Soviet soldiers believe that neither ideology nor political indoctrination is very effective in producing a genuine state of reflexive conditioning. Soviet soldiers were asked: "Among the soldiers that you knew, do you think that classes in political subjects and ideology were important in making a soldier want to be a good soldier?" Of the 103 former Soviet soldiers responding, only 20.4 percent agreed that such classes were an important motivator; 75.2 percent indicated that such factors as ideology were not very important.[5] If the data are examined a bit further and we ask how important a soldier's belief in Marxist-Leninism was in motivating him to fight well, it appears that the data do not support the view that the social conditioning of the Soviet soldier is having much impact. The data shown in Table 1 are self-explanatory and suggest that for most Soviet soldiers, ideology per se is not having the impact on behavior needed to develop the conditioned reflex that Soviet psychiatry says it can develop.[6] The data suggest, at least tentatively, that the Soviet soldier does not regard either ideology or his exposure to political indoctrination classes as important motivators for his military behavior.

Table 1
Perception of Ideology as an Important Factor in Motivation

"Among the soldiers that you knew, do you think that classes in political subjects and ideology are important in making a soldier want to be a good soldier?"

	Number	Percent
Yes	23	20.4
No	85	75.2

N = 103

Excluded: 5

Richard A. Gabriel, *The Mind of the Soviet Fighting Man* (Westport, Conn.: Greenwood Press, 1984), p. 30.

If ideology is not a strong motivating force, then what does motivate the Soviet soldier? Again, the data must be approached with caution. When Soviet soldiers were asked what things were the most important to motivating the soldier to fight well, they listed "not wanting to appear a coward in front of your friends" as the most important reason for fighting well.[7] (See Table 2.) By contrast, they listed a belief in ideology at a much lower level, suggesting once again that ideology is simply not sufficiently rooted in the mind of the Soviet fighting man to serve as a trigger for a truly conditioned reflex that would determine behavior.

Table 2
Important Factors in Fighting Spirit

"Which of the following things do you think is most important in motivating a soldier to fight well?"

	Number	Percent
Close ties to his comrades in the unit	23	20.4
Support of one's friends back home	19	16.8
Feeling that one's officers and NCOs care about you	5	4.4
Belief in an ideology	12	10.6
Not wanting to appear a coward in front of your friends	50	44.2
N = 109		
	Excluded: 4	

Gabriel, *Mind of the Soviet Fighting Man*, p. 30.

If this tentative and incomplete evidence can be said to at least partially reflect the peacetime attitude structure of most Soviet soldiers, then it appears that, although the social conditioning of the Soviet soldier in terms of his exposure to the state's official ideology does form an important background variable as Donnelly suggests, in terms of actually motivating military behavior, other factors are apparently far more important. Many of these are the same as those found in Western armies, namely, the importance of strong social ties, the respect of one's peers, trust in one's leaders, and so on. These factors, even for the Soviet soldier, seem to be more important motivators than Marxist-Leninist ideology.

MILITARY TRAINING

The Soviet Army, like all armies, places great emphasis on realistic training to guard against battle stress. A considerable body of data suggests, however, that training per se is not decisive. Dr. David Marlowe of the Walter Reed Army Institute of Research in Washington, D.C., has observed that the rate of psychiatric breakdown due to battlefield stress is similar among veteran soldiers and new soldiers over time.[8] Nonetheless, the Soviets place a great premium on realistic battle training because they believe that the individual is essentially a physiological organism that reacts fundamentally to objective stimuli expressed in terms of what the organism has been oriented to expect. Put another way, to the extent that the soldier can be acclimated to an environment that approximates actual combat, then the organism's responses to these events will be conditioned so that it will respond in the way it has been trained. Thus, "the main purpose of training is to mold in the serviceman the qualities which enable him to carry out any combat mission, to act courageously and resolute under conditions of increased danger, to control their behavior in battle and to endure high physical loads of psychological stress."[9] Soviet military training is designed to condition the soldier to "know" the conditions of war and to inculcate in him a patterned response by teaching him to respond to specific stimuli. Soviet training is geared as much to teaching the soldier to endure stress as it is to teach him military skills. In the West, the training emphasis is on the soldier's skills. In practice, the Soviet emphasis is on strict obedience to orders as a response to predictable circumstances. As with so much of Soviet military psychiatry, Soviet training doctrine is based on the Pavlovian notion of orienting responses to external stimuli.

The Soviets train their soldiers to a demanding physical regimen and to specific tasks. Soviet military psychiatrists train the soldier to perform a specific set of tasks under specified conditions to which he is expected to respond when confronted by the reality of battle. Thus, under conditions of stress, the soldier is expected to keep control if he is properly trained and if the conditions under which he was trained (objective reality) are approximated in battle. Even if the excitation in the brain is strong enough to disrupt his conscious thinking processes, he may be "literally taken in hand" by those conditioned reflexes learned in training and perform anyway. The inculcation of these reflexes makes it "possible in spite of the confusion to maintain a correct direction of the rhythm of his actions." In short, the soldier's reactions can be automatic, if not conscious. Although Westerners may think that strange, the fact is that the British Army practiced a primitive variant of this same idea during the early Afghan wars in the nineteenth century through a practice called "pokey drill."

In pokey drill blindfolded soldiers practiced loading and unloading their bolt action Martini rifles with wooden cartridges. The point of the exercise, which was often repeated for hours on end, was that the soldier could be made to perform certain basic tasks so automatically that, when he came under fire and his conscious thinking processes were disrupted, he could still continue to execute his task. Most Western armies have abandoned this philosophy of training because it is held to be dangerous for a soldier to suspend his thinking processes. Although an individual can be taught to respond almost automatically to comparatively simple tasks, in general, the level of complexity of the tasks that can be learned and accomplished in this manner is very limited.

The Western experience has been that rote training does not work. The Soviets, on the other hand, have reduced their training programs to a level where the soldier is required to perform only four or five specific tasks, to do them well and on cue, and to be reliable in doing them. There is no such thing in the Soviet Army as a secondary MOS (military operational specialty) or cross training, at least not to the extent that one finds them in the West. The Soviet soldier is expected to perform only a few simple tasks, but to perform them under the most arduous circumstances. Basically, he is expected to stand and fight and to fire his weapon regardless of the horror around him. Soviet training doctrine, while harsh, is also very simple, which is advantageous in times of stress when the soldier's ability to make decisions is reduced in any case. By keeping the soldier's expectations simple, by requiring that he perform the same tasks, and by making him continually respond to the same stimuli over and over again, the Soviets hope to build a soldier who is highly resistant to battle stress breakdown.

In their military training, the Soviets do not seek to train a soldier to make decisions under stress. Quite the contrary. Rather, they attempt to create a conditioned response based on Marxist-Leninist and Pavlovian ideas of human psychology which will all but obviate the need for individual decisions. Yet, that this kind of "deep" conditioning can be achieved in so short a training period as that available to the Soviet Army is problematical. With two years of constant training, the Soviet soldier will likely become relatively proficient in the application of his military skills. But whether the level of skill can be raised to the point where Soviet military psychiatrists would consider it to be a genuine conditioned reflex rooted in the physiology of the brain and the second signal system remains, at best, unproven. Western psychiatrists believe that a genuine conditioned response cannot be formed without much more time and much more intensive exposure to stimuli. Neither Soviet military training nor any other kind of training, given the conditions under which it must operate, is probably sufficiently thorough, repetitive or intensive to create a genuine conditioned reflex.

Although one can condition a person to any number of biological reflexes, it remains unclear as to whether the principles of conditioning can meaningfully be applied to the higher mental activity of the human being. Furthermore, anyone familiar with Soviet training understands that training schedules and practice confront at least the same problems encountered in Western armies. For example, the Soviet press often bemoans the substandard quality of training. Soviet military periodicals frequently point out that military training is simplistic. This is a chronic problem in all armies. Unrealistic training is perhaps more the norm than the exception in all armies, and the Soviet Army seems to be no exception. When practical problems of supply, crossing bridges, blowing up houses, or other training activities present themselves, military trainers often solve them "administratively," that is, they certify that certain things have been done when they have not. It may be practical for a training officer to "simulate" an artillery barrage on a platoon, but such a simulation can hardly be expected to condition the troops to the real thing when they face it. In addition, all armies must endure what the Soviets call the problem of slackening in training. As in

Western armies, this means that there is almost always insufficient time and money to conduct thorough training. Moreover, the troops often have other things to do besides training, not the least of which, in the Soviet case, is attending political classes. Thus, if the object of training is to create within the soldier a conditioned pattern of response to battlefield stimuli, it seems that Soviet military training is inadequate to generate the conditions Soviet military psychiatrists assert is the purpose of training.

When Soviet soldiers were asked to assess the quality of their training, they generally tended to rate it fairly high. As Table 3 shows, Soviet soldiers who were asked to rate the quality of their military training on a scale from one to ten generally gave it good marks, with the mean being 5.5.[10] American soldiers responded much the same way when asked the same question. Perhaps more importantly, when Soviet soldiers were asked to relate the quality of their military training to their ability to perform in combat, they generally gave their units high marks. (See Table 4.)

Table 3
Perceived Quality of Soviet Military Training

"On a scale of from one to ten in which one is the worst and ten is the best how would you rate the military training that your unit received?"

	Number	Percent
1	6	5.3
2	8	7.1
3	14	12.4
4	9	8.0
5	20	17.7
6	7	6.2
7	18	15.9
8	16	14.2
9	3	2.7
10	7	6.2

N = 113

Median score: 5.5

Gabriel, *Mind of the Soviet Fighting Man*, p. 12.

When Soviet soldiers were asked, "In your opinion how well do you think your unit would fight in actual combat," nearly half the soldiers believed that their units would have fought very well or fairly well. Only a small number, under 16 percent, regarded their troop training as producing poor or very poor units.[11] These data tend to parallel fairly closely the findings of the American Army and other Western armies when similar questions are asked of their soldiers (see Gabriel, *The Antagonists: A Comparative Combat Assessment of the Soviet and American Soldier*, Greenwood, 1983).

Table 4
Perceptions Rating Combat Ability of Soviet Units

"In your opinion how well do you think your unit would have fought in actual combat?"

	Number	Percent
Very well	10	8.6
Fairly well	41	36.4
Moderately well	38	33.6
Poorly	16	14.2
Very poorly	2	1.8

N = 107

Excluded: 6

Gabriel, *Mind of the Soviet Fighting Man*, p. 13.

There is no evidence then, that the quality of Soviet military training, which may be better or worse than military training in the West, is, in itself, sufficient to produce a conditioned reflex in the soldier so strong and so embedded that he will become immunized against battlefield stress. On the other hand, Soviet soldiers are generally well trained and are, therefore, likely to perform better in battle, although, in fact, their susceptibility to stress breakdown may be no more or less than that of untrained troops over time. The training of the Soviet soldier can only be seen as fulfilling the requirements of Soviet military psychiatry for the development of a conditioned reflex in the most marginal sense. It does not seem to be more successful in this area than Western military training.

The Soviet military also uses simplistic battle drills in its battle stress programs. The Soviets are acutely aware that, under stress, one of the mental abilities that decays first and most rapidly is the ability to process information and make decisions. What remains is his ability to react precisely in the way he has been trained, and the simpler the task he is expected to carry out the more likely he will be able to do so. Accordingly, they play down the idea of individual initiative which, in any case, they regard derogatively as "native wit," a trait they associate with peasant cunning and the peasant's tendency to avoid responsibilities.[12] Instead, under the Soviet military system all plans for doctrinal and strategic applications are made in advance and are then carried out with a burst of intensive activity until the objectives are obtained. In contrast, in the West, individuals and units are expected to be able to adapt rapidly to changing battlefield conditions. The Soviets seem convinced that, under conditions of great stress, the army that has planned to execute a particular maneuver and rigidly adheres to that plan is likely to carry the day even if the cost in lives is very high.

This difference in military doctrine and its emphasis on conditioning the soldier against stress arises from historical differences between Russian and Western doctrine. Three factors strongly influenced the development of Soviet doctrine.[13] First is the geographic size of the Russian homeland, which is much greater than that of any other European country in which a war was ever fought. The Soviets have had to sustain large armies and maneuver them in a controlled manner. In the West, the emphasis has been on the creation and use of relatively small units and their adjustment to continually changing circumstances. The second is the nature of the terrain which has affected Soviet military thought to a great degree. In Western Europe, the terrain is hilly and marked by rivers, forests, and large urban concentrations that can be used to strategic or tactical advantage. In the Soviet Union, the terrain is essentially flat and open, and is far more like a sea or naked desert in its tactical applications. As a result, Western armies have developed the concept of using the terrain to great advantage. Russian terrain presents the military planner with quite a different problem, namely, how to concentrate forces quickly, move them about in exposed positions, and close rapidly with the enemy before he has a chance to destroy one's forces in the open. (The Soviet penchant for large concentrations of long-range artillery guns is one solution to this problem.) This means that the doctrine of using minimal applications of force while taking greatest advantage of the terrain, which rests at the base of Western tactical thought, never received serious attention in the Soviet Union. The tactical problem for the Soviet field commander has historically been fundamentally different in that he must be able to concentrate large units that can move long distances and still be able to close rapidly with the enemy and destroy him. This has placed a premium not on initiative and use of terrain but on control and ensuring that large units and their subcomponents behave according to plan.

The third factor is the low population density of the country and its relatively sparse communications networks. As a consequence, the Soviets have been forced to stress the control and maneuver of large units and simplicity as the only way to move large forces across vast areas of open country efficiently. Unlike Western terrain where armies could hole up in and draw sustenance from a number of cities or other resource centers like ports and railheads, in the Soviet Union such facilities have been historically rare or thinly dispersed over great distances. Therefore, Soviet military thought focuses on making large armies self-sustaining for long periods and able to operate under arduous conditions of shortages. Recall, for example, that Soviet divisions in World War II normally went into battle at only 75 percent strength in manpower and equipment. These three factors have meant that the battle conditions under which the Soviet soldier has been expected to fight have been considerably more rigorous than in the West—so much so that considerations of minor tactical details have been subordinated to the need to mass large units, move them quickly, and hammer the enemy even at the expense of great casualties.

This last difference in Soviet and Western tactical doctrines is evident in the Soviet willingness to absorb enormous numbers of casualties in order to achieve tactical and strategic objectives. In World War II, the Soviet Army lost far more men than any other combatant and fought under conditions of terrible hardship. Unit for unit, the German Army probably outfought the Soviets, and, generally, German officers were far superior to Soviet officers. But, in the end, the ability to concentrate large battle formations, to mass large numbers of tanks and artillery guns, and to take the offensive and overwhelm the enemy, if only in a sea of numbers, proved decisive. For the Soviets, the question was not so much how they fought the war but whether or not they won the war. All evidence that the Germans outfought them, outgeneralled them, and were better at tactics counted for nothing in the end.

The Soviets contend that the overall system is the most important influence in enabling the soldier to resist stress breakdown. The key, according to the Soviets, is to formulate military plans at the highest level, usually at army or front level, and then to restrict the initiative of the lower level commanders in the implementation of the plan. This restriction removes the necessity of decision-making under stress. In the Soviet Army, no plans are made below division. Division-size units as well as units within the division are expected to execute precisely the plans formulated by higher headquarters. The relationship between a Soviet army and a division in terms of decision-making is about the same as that between an American division and a battalion. The Soviets deliberately restrict the options of lower unit commanders so that they will have fewer choices to make under stress.

Soviet doctrine also emphasizes the ability to deliver shock, attain surprise, concentrate mass, and take the offensive, all of which, in Western thought, tend to reduce stress casualties. Psychiatric casualties are normally greater in defensive than in offensive actions and always greater when units are taken by surprise than when they inflict surprise. Western research also shows that stress casualties are greater under conditions of indirect fire and of greater complexity.

Taken together, the ability of Soviet units to develop a rigid plan, to rest and build up their forces for the attack, and then to implement it with a great deal of shock, ferocity, and surprise, accompanied by massive concentrations of air and artillery fire delivered by indirect fire weapons, helps increase the probabilities of paralyzing the will of the defender while at the same time reducing the attacker's psychiatric casualties. The Soviets have drawn a clear connection between the way battle drills are executed, the way the command and control structure of military units work, and the way these factors help reduce the stress placed on the soldier in battle. In principle, if a soldier can always take the offensive, inflict shock against the enemy, possess the element of surprise, have a preponderance of fire, and relentlessly press the assault, then these conditions, in and of themselves, will reduce the level of psychiatric casualties that will be suffered by Soviet units. The reverse of these conditions will produce large numbers of battle stress casualties. The Soviets seem to have drawn these conclusions from their detailed studies of battlefield performance in World War II, and have adjusted their military structure and doctrine accordingly. They believe that the use of these basic battle doctrines will significantly reduce psychiatric casualties.

Everything about the Soviet military in battle is simplified: their choice of tactics, their resupply of forces, and even their design of fighting vehicles and weapons. Simplicity is the key. This is evident even in the initiative granted the Soviet commander. When a Soviet commander is told to exercise "initiative," this does not mean that he is to devise a plan for changing battlefield conditions and react accordingly. Rather, Soviet commanders are trained to execute a limited range of eight to ten basic battle drills. When the Soviet commander is asked to exercise initiative, he is really being asked to make a choice among these few battle drills and to apply the drill that is most likely to succeed or accommodate the circumstances he faces. In contrast, initiative for the Western soldier means developing completely new solutions to fundamentally unforeseen problems.

The Soviets have also greatly simplified their logistical structure. Basically, the Soviet logistical system is a "push" system as opposed to the "pull" system that characterizes the American Army. Soviet logisticians have calculated scientifically and algorithmically the rates at which certain stocks will be depleted under certain battle conditions. They then stock the number and type of supplies relative to the type of battle, and they continue to push supplies forward to the attacking units rather than waiting for these units to deplete their supplies and request replacements. As such, the whole supply system is much simpler than the systems usually found in Western armies; for the Soviets, this simplicity facilitates military effectiveness and, coincidentally, reduces stress casualties.

Yet another area in which simplicity is evident is in military equipment design. Anyone who has studied Soviet military equipment closely, whether the AK–47 assault rifle or the T–72 main battle tank, understands that the Soviets only rarely make radical design departures from previous equipment models. The more common approach is to modify existing equipment, making small changes and thereby gradually developing the design until it can meet new battlefield requirements. The reason is to keep things simple and to ensure that the soldier knows precisely what his tasks are. It is quite possible to take a Soviet reservist who has been out of active military service for five years and put him in the new T–72 battle tank and have him find it just as easy to drive and similar in layout to the T–62 he may have trained on five years earlier. It is highly unlikely that his American counterpart could operate the new M–1 tank or fire the new generation of missiles that has come into the inventory. Therefore, the doctrine of simplicity is a major characteristic of Soviet tactics, logistics, and equipment design.

The Soviets have developed battle drills for maximizing the impact of stress on the enemy by using speed of maneuver, concentration of effort, and the attainment of surprise. The Soviet commander's objective is not to grind the enemy down by a war of attrition, a common misconception of Soviet tactics in World War II held in the West. Rather, it is to deliver the enemy a shock to his entire military system, with a very heavy initial blow followed by a rapid advance deep into his rear. The object is to paralyze the enemy in the attack and leave him unable to act. The Soviets use shock as a major mechanism for incapacitating the enemy's entire military system, much as shock can be used to incapacitate the individual soldier.

The Soviets have made detailed studies of the impact of certain weapons on the ability of the enemy to maintain psychological stability. In this area they seem to be quite far ahead of the West. Their research findings have been incorporated into their military manuals so that a commander will know that certain weapons at his disposal have predictable psychological effects on the enemy. If employed correctly, such weapons will reduce the enemy's ability to resist precisely because they will induce specified levels of psychological shock. Hence, the Soviet military has tried to estimate the degree to which the enemy will suffer psychological incapacitation due to shock. For example, if a Soviet regiment in the attack fires one unit of its artillery supply, approximately 600 rounds, Soviet manuals calculate that although only 25 percent of the defenders will be killed or wounded by blast effects, almost 90 percent of the defenders will be incapacitated for several minutes as a result of psychological shock. In another case, an enemy machine gunner subjected to one unit of artillery fire from a regiment will be unable to operate his weapon for 3.5 minutes; a truck driver will be unable to operate his vehicle for seven minutes; or a fire direction center will be unable to direct fire for eleven minutes; and so on. In short, the Soviets have not only utilized their doctrinal and tactical thinking to immunize their own soldiers against stress, but have also turned the problem around so that they can calculate the impact of stress on the specific military operational skills of the enemy soldier. In this sense, they have fully integrated the findings of military psychiatry into their combat operations. They intend to use this information to good effect by employing combat pulses of great ferocity in pursuit of battlefield objectives, regardless of the casualties suffered. This is how the Soviet Army fought World War II, and it is how they intend to fight the next war.

BATTLE DISCIPLINE

The Soviets employ a rigid disciplinary code in dealing with battle stress. The discipline of the Soviet military on the battlefield is probably more severe than that of all modern Western armies—if not in its cruelty, then at least in its rigor and thoroughness. In World War II no fewer than 250 general officers were executed or sent to penal battalions for failing to demonstrate sufficient courage in the face of the enemy.[14] With regard to the common soldier, execution of a soldier or officer in front of his unit was regarded as company punishment that required no formal legal procedure to implement. In addition, extensive use was made of penal battalions to which soldiers who had committed crimes or who had not been resolute enough in battle were sent. Life in the penal battalions was extremely harsh. The battalions were often employed on suicide missions and suffered staggeringly high casualties. The Soviet view of harsh battlefield discipline evolved not only from its military experience, but also from its political experience. It must be remembered that the USSR has a long history of using absolute power and of not trusting its citizenry or its soldiers. Discipline is regarded as absolutely necessary to get soldiers to perform in a way they would not otherwise wish to do.

With regard to reducing stress, Soviet psychiatric theory has always advocated the use of harsh discipline of which the soldier is made well aware in advance of his military training. As discussed earlier, the Soviets believe that resistance to stress is possible when the individual is properly oriented to his environment. A soldier must be cognizant not only of the conditions under which he must perform, but also of the penalties for failure to perform. Both are equally compelling stimuli in guiding human behavior. A key concept in Soviet theory is the dynamic stereotype, an idea that implies that the organism must come to know that he has a choice between two types of action. Down one path lies an almost certain death, namely, execution for cowardice, or at least very harsh treatment in the penal battalion where he may lose his life anyway. Down the other path lies at least the possibility of honor and survival. The Soviets believe strongly that part of conditioning the soldier to perform correctly under stress is to buttress his positive conditioning with the threat of strong punishments for failure.

The Soviet disciplinary system does not rely entirely on negative means such as execution or imprisonment. Equally important is the role of the political officer. Unlike any army in the West, the Soviet Army has an officer in every company, battalion, regiment, and division who is in charge of the morale, motivation, and ideological consciousness of the soldiers in the unit. The political officer helps to motivate the soldier, a task he often accomplishes by holding political classes, acting as a counselor and even as a friend. The Soviet disciplinary system is balanced in its severity by placing an officer in the combat units whose job is to monitor and develop combat spirit, motivation, and morale. The record of World War II suggests that, in many instances, the political officer was the key to maintaining a unit's fighting spirit.

Soviet standards of battlefield discipline are severe by Western standards. Western armies are ruled by the presumption that concerns of larger patriotism motivate the soldier to fight, although the feelings of cohesion that result from the strong, mutually supportive human relationships within units contribute most to fighting spirit. The West, therefore, maintains that there are clear limits beyond which one cannot force a soldier to perform. In contrast, at no level does the Soviet military operate by self-motivation. Despite the great efforts made to motivate the soldier, fundamentally the Soviet military is a "driven" system that relies heavily on strong discipline to buttress whatever ideological or patriotic concerns the soldier himself may consider important. In the final analysis, the Soviets regard the soldier much the same way the regime regards the citizen and certainly much as the czars regarded the peasantry. There is a basic feeling that generally life is difficult and that life in the military is even more so, and that, all things being equal, the soldier will try to escape whatever hardships the military will impose on him, particularly battle. The Soviets are not embarrassed to admit that despite all the propaganda, all the conditioning, all the psychological training to steel the soldier's will, if all else fails, harsh discipline will compel the soldier to perform as expected, or it will extract his life as the cost of failure. This view is unacceptable in modern Western armies (although at one time it was, as in World War I). But this system has worked well historically for the Soviets, and so they have great confidence in it. It is unlikely to change in the near future.

DRUGS

Although some Soviet publications have raised the possibility of using drugs in conditioning the soldier against battle stress, insufficient information is available to document the details of drug applications in this form. The Soviets are probably continuing research into the use of chemical agents in conditioning (and conversations with present and former Soviet psychiatrists confirm this), but the exact details remain sketchy. Drug production and even experimentation with drug compounds is relatively new in the Soviet Union. Both before and during World War II, the Soviets made substantial use of folk and herb medicines for the treatment of disease, including psychiatric casualties, but their drug industry lagged behind that of the West. Among the reasons for this situation was the disruption and destruction caused by World War II. Only now, in the last fifteen years, has the USSR begun to catch up to the West in the production of drugs. But in terms of the variety and purity of drug production, the Soviet drug industry is still behind.

Interviews with Soviet psychiatrists as well as medical doctors and pharmacologists reveal that drug purity and refinement in the

Soviet Union is poor. The drugs often produce a number of unwanted, and even paradoxical, side effects. As a consequence, many of the tranquilizers and stimulants used are imported, West Germany and France being the two largest sources of imported drugs from the West and East Germany and Hungary from Eastern Europe. By Western standards, the Soviet drug industry is still relatively primitive, but the clinical application of drugs is quite advanced and new drugs reach the clinical marketplace much faster than in the United States.

Soviet technical literature has high praise for the potential uses of psychostimulators and tranquilizers. This literature notes that psychostimulators can be used to "eliminate the sense of fatigue and elevate the intellectual and physical working capability while having an antihypnotic effect and facilitating the elevation of mood. These hold an important place in the series of physiological agents capable of compensating for the psychological disadaptation in the borderline states."[15] The Soviets are, of course, seriously exploring drugs as a mechanism for conditioning, given their physiological assumptions regarding human behavior.

In terms of psychostimulants, Soviet technical literature reveals the following positive effects aiding the soldier in coping with battle stress: (1) the activation of intellectual activity, which helps the mind to process information; (2) acceleration of the thinking and speaking process; (3) mild euphoria; (4) increased activity and temporary elimination of fatigue; and (5) stimulation of alertness and decrease in appetite.[16] The chemical stimulants range from artificial compounds to natural stimulants such as caffeine, alcohol, and extract of magnolia vine.

Soviet psychiatrists are clearly interested in the military applications of psychostimulants and tranquilizers, but a survey of twenty years of Soviet medical literature reveals only a handful of publicized applications of research dealing with military uses for drugs and battlefield behavior. And the few studies that are available are relatively recent. Even more recent is the research on improving the soldier's physical performance through drugs and autosuggestion. For years the Soviets have given preeminence to political training and other forms of conditioning against stress. Only within the last decade has there been any work detailing actual clinical applications in the use of drugs and battlefield stress.

A small list of drugs that appear in Soviet medical literature have military applications. The degree of military application, however, remains in question. The Soviets are probably still in the testing stages and are using them essentially in clinical research settings. No hard evidence exists of any widespread practical applications of psychostimulants and other drugs in battle.

Some of the drugs mentioned in the technical literature which have potential military applications include phenamine (amphetamine sulfate) which was used in World War II. This drug appears to be the first psychostimulant the Soviets used in order to increase battlefield performance, and it may still be in use today. Its effect is to produce a short-term burst of energy, but it is often accompanied by highly paradoxical side effects and causes exhaustion. Another drug is penatine, a combination of phenamine and nicotine, and it is also used as a stimulant. It was used in 1969 in a series of small experiments with artillery gunners in order to determine how long gunners could continue to fire while under the influence of the stimulant. Ostensibly, its effects are milder than phenamine alone without producing addiction or severe exhaustion.

A third drug is syndocarb, a general but strong stimulant that may be somewhat better than amphetamine. Because it is a stronger compound, the Soviets feel it is easier to target the drug against specific symptoms. In addition, relative to amphetamine its action is more gradual, so that there is no "rush" of excitement, and its effects are longer lasting. Syndocarb seems to be unaccompanied by either euphoria or motor excitation and, apparently, has only limited side effects such as muscle weakness or inability to sleep.

Two other drugs that appear in Soviet literature are phenaput and trioxizine. Phenaput is a broad spectrum tranquilizer, probably not akin to valium or any other benzodiazephine, and is a derivative of GABA (gamma amino buteric acid). Trioxizine is also a tranquilizer with identifiable properties like librium. Phenaput was used in military experiments as early as 1970 by L. I. Spivak before he became chief of the Department of Psychiatry at the Kirov Military Medical Academy. In the experiments, an attempt was made to reduce stress among paratroopers and riflemen by administering the drug to them over a twenty-day period and measuring the differences in their ability to hit rifle targets. Phenaput may also be used to reduce fear and extend motor activity. The Soviets used this drug during the American-Soviet space link-up with *Soyuz*.

In assessing the effectiveness of drug applications as a means of combating stress, it seems fair to suggest that the Soviets are probably no further advanced in their research than is the West. In fact, they may be considerably behind Western research efforts. More importantly, whatever military applications the Soviets may have developed have been restricted to small research projects. There is absolutely no evidence of any widespread use of either tranquilizers or psychostimulants as preventatives or as immunizers of stress within the military. As we will see later, the Soviets employ a wide range of drugs in treating battle stress, but as a prophylactic, the Soviets have made little progress in dealing with chemical therapies for stress. Given the physiological orientation of Soviet military psychiatry, it seems only logical that they will put significant effort into finding chemical means to increase the efficiency of the physiological mechanisms which they see as conditioning human behavior.

In conclusion, the Soviets are apparently giving the problem of battle stress a lot of attention. This attention dates back to only 1967, when the Soviets decided that large-scale conventional operations were possible after all even in a nuclear environment. As physiologists, they have done a considerable amount of work on how the nuclear battlefield would disrupt the soldier's mental patterns. They have approached the problem of battleshock in a serious and systematic manner and have developed several programs to deal with it.

In Soviet psychiatric theory, these immunizing processes are designed not only to reduce the level of combat stress, but also to develop a physiologically defined conditioned reflex in the mind of the soldier. Experience in the West suggests that this kind of reflex pattern can be created only within the confines of a laboratory. The capacity to condition an individual to respond to a specific stimulus under stress, especially in circumstances that involve the higher mental processes, is much more difficult to achieve (if it is achievable at all) than is granted by Soviet psychiatric theory.

The Soviet experience in World War II has taught them that the soldier who is convinced of the moral superiority of his cause, and who is given rigorous training, taught simple battle drills, and strict battlefield discipline, is less likely to become a stress casualty in the first place. Furthermore, a harsh definition of the symptoms that allow a soldier out of combat precludes the development of a number of symptomologies that are acceptable in the West. The cultural values that determine acceptable behavior will further determine what kind of behavior finally emerges under fire, particularly with regard to psychiatric adjustments to stressful situations. The empirical impact of drugs on this equation is too new in the Soviet case (as in the West) to assess with any accuracy.

Soviet psychiatric theory notwithstanding, battleshock casualties appear inevitable in all armies under conditions of great stress. Although their rates, degree of treatment, rates of recovery, and types of treatment may vary, the fact that soldiers will break down under conditions of war seems a fact of military life. And it is fast becoming a major problem as the killing power of weaponry increases almost exponentially. The critical factor in determining how much manpower will eventually be lost to psychiatric causes seems to depend on how such casualties are diagnosed and treated when they occur. Because they cannot reasonably be prevented in their totality, it is important to ask how the modern Soviet military medical structure is geared to handling battle stress casualties.

6
Soviet Battlefield Psychiatry

This chapter examines the structure and practice of modern Soviet battle psychiatry. The analysis centers on the approach of Western military psychiatrists, and an attempt is made to discern the counterpart functions performed by Soviet military psychiatrists.

One major task of military psychiatrists in Western armies is to screen conscripts for military service. During World War II, the U.S. military developed extensive screening mechanisms for sorting out the conscripts with questionable ability to withstand the stress of combat. The standard for both psychiatric and physical fitness was the same, namely, that all soldiers who entered military service were expected to be "fit for combat." Almost no thought was given, at least until 1944, to selecting conscripts who were not fit to withstand battle but who could be used in noncombat assignments. As a consequence, psychiatric screening eliminated a great deal of manpower that could otherwise have been put to good use in support, supply, and administrative roles. This was not the case for the Soviet Army in World War II, and it is not the case now.

As discussed earlier in this book, during World War II, the Soviets examined approximately 22 million conscripts for military service. Fewer than 100,000 (and perhaps fewer than 75,000) were rejected for purely psychiatric reasons.[1] No exemptions or releases were granted for "unsuitability" or "failure to adapt" as was commonly the case in the American Army. Moreover, in terms of physical rejections, perhaps no more than 250,000 conscripts were rejected for physical reasons. Although conscripts were given standard military physical examinations that focused on finding any debilitating diseases of the heart, lungs, circulatory system, nutritional problems, and other basic categories of physical weakness, the fact remains that less than 1 percent of all Soviet conscripts were rejected for military service for these reasons. In a practical sense, the Soviet Army impressed almost every conscript it examined.

With regard to draft screening today, the Soviet military psychiatrist has a much smaller role than his counterpart in the West and, in many cases, the role is practically nonexistent. In dealing with conscripts who might manifest psychiatric problems, a Soviet draft board (draft commissariat) is provided with a list of all patients who are undergoing psychiatric care within the relevant military district. The civilian public health system is structurally parallel to the military district and commissariat system used for conscription. If the civilian health clinic diagnoses the conscript as having a serious problem or a history of psychiatric illness, the military usually does not even call the conscript in for an examination. Those with marginal or recent histories of mental disturbances are usually called and examined by the usual team of military doctors comprised of internists and neurologists. Sometimes a psychiatrist takes extra time to determine if a conscript is faking. Soldiers without any mental history are given perfunctory neurologic examinations rather similar to those given to U.S. conscripts. There is no battery of psychiatric tests administered to conscripts by psychiatrists. Nor does there appear to be any systematic use of psychiatric questionnaires. In general, if the conscript has not established a history of mental illness prior to being called for military service, the military will make every effort to ensure that he serves.

Every civilian health district within the Soviet Union has a neuropsychiatric dispensary that keeps records on all patients within the district with psychotic or severe neurotic mental health problems. The structure of the mental health clinics was established in the mid–1920s. In the mid–1970s, the Ministry of Mental Health and the Institute of Forensic Psychiatry established a project to computerize all information on every patient in the country who had been treated within the public health system, with special emphasis on psychiatric conditions. A centralized computer file is now kept on all psychiatric patients. The basic diagnostic categories used by the Soviets to categorize the data are those used by ICD–9, the commonly recognized international diagnostic manual widely used in the West. An effort is also made to enforce these diagnostic categories on psychiatric practitioners within the district and dispensary hospitals as a way of imposing some unity on the diagnostic criteria used by the civilian and military authorities in dealing with psychiatric cases. The goal is to develop a common diagnostic terminology that will be functional for both sets of authorities.

In 1980, the Institute for Forensic Psychiatry conducted a study of the military's psychiatric screening procedures as well as the basic psychiatric applications of the national public health system. They discovered two interesting facts. First, on a nationwide basis the level of diagnosed cases of schizophrenia in each mental health district tended to vary directly with the number of psychiatrists who were present within each mental health district. The greater the number of psychiatrists present in each district, the greater the number of diagnosed cases of schizophrenia. Second, in their study of draft rejections for psychiatric reasons, the institute found that the highest rates of draft rejections for psychiatric reasons were in the Baltic republics of Latvia, Estonia, and Lithuania.[2] The highest rate was in Lithuania where the rejection rate was eight times higher than for any other Soviet republic. The most common diagnostic reason for these rejections was oligophrenia which, in the Soviet lexicon, may be generally translated as mental retardation or "dullwittedness." Lest such a diagnostic category seem strange to the Western mind, it is useful to recall that in World War I, one of the most common causes of rejection in the American Army was for a similar condition then defined as "imbecillia."

Soviet authorities saw a functional connection between the number of psychiatrists and the rate of mental illness diagnosed in both the public health and military conscript examining systems. They also suspected a conspiracy among the Baltic republics to exempt their citizens from military service. Although nothing is known about what Soviet authorities did to correct these problems, the study did reinforce a basic premise of Soviet psychiatric medicine. Since World War II, the Soviets have assumed that the presence of psychiatrists would in itself increase the frequency of diagnosed mental problems among the troops. Indeed, they have assumed that the presence of any medical doctor would increase the number of medical complaints generated by the soldiery and, worse, that it would also increase the number of soldiers who as a result would be temporarily removed from duty. Soviet military psychiatrists often cite these facts when they try to explain why the Soviet Army does not employ psychiatrists at the division level or below. The Israeli experience in the 1982 Lebanon war seems to tentatively confirm the Soviet position: In the Israeli experience of 1982, as many as one-third of their casualties may have been due to improper diagnosis.

With regard to draft avoidance or duty assignments based on psychiatric disability, Soviet military authorities assume as a matter of course that a sizable number of people will attempt to fake mental or physical problems as a way of escaping the rigors of military service. They assume, as Russian authorities have always assumed, that the citizenry will often have to be forced to do unpleasant things. As noted earlier, the Soviet military system is not based on self-motivation, despite the general belief that the soldier can be motivated by ideological conviction. It is, a "driven system" in which individuals are forced to do what they would normally not do. As in any army, Soviet conscripts use a number of tricks to escape military service. But the Soviet examiners' emphasis on physiological disability as opposed to psychiatric disability has made the task of the reluctant conscript very difficult. Such ruses as placing pencil lead under one's tongue to produce a fever or taking drugs or binging on sugar in order to produce physical symptoms of illness are not uncommon, but they do appear to be far less effective in eliminating the conscript from military service than in some countries in the West.

In order to deal with the inventiveness of conscripts, Soviet doctors often segregate soldiers with specific symptoms that appear to be false or self-induced. Soviet doctors generally treat the symptoms in such a way as to make the complaints worse. In one instance, for example, soldiers who were complaining of diarrhea were given stool softeners for three days, the theory being that if they were faking to begin with, the discomfort of having to defecate all the time was worse than submitting to their military duties. With such an approach to military medicine, it might be expected that Soviet units have fewer "sick book riders" in their ranks than in armies of the West. Reporting ill is, in most instances, not a very effective way to avoid military duties.

As in all armies, attempts to avoid military service and medical complaints are tolerated to a degree. But if a soldier complains too often, or attempts to avoid duty or service with a false medical complaint, he can be charged with the crime of malingering, and the punishment can be harsh. On balance, however, the level of medical complaints and attempts to avoid service has not been significant for the Soviet Army since 1967 when the Soviets established a nationwide system of premilitary training and physical screening. And, too, as discussed earlier, the medical examiners' narrow view of psychiatric problems has reduced the problem of draft and duty avoidance. Problems that might qualify an individual for rejection in Western armies—such as mild neurosis, anxiety, night sweats, or bed wetting—are not acceptable in the Soviet Army. Rather, they are seen as reflecting a lack of character or a defective personality which the conscript has a responsibility to overcome.

With the establishment of DOSAAF in 1967, the already low rate of exemption for psychiatric reasons dropped even further. Unlike his Western counterpart, a Soviet conscript reports to his military commissariat for draft examination with a long and detailed history involving not only medical aspects, but social and educational aspects as well. All Soviet youth between the ages of sixteen and seventeen are enrolled in the DOSAAF system where they undergo military training and physical conditioning. Extensive records are kept on their behavior and attitudes. This file precedes the conscript to the draft commissariat even before he is called to military service. As such, a conscript with a record of normal behavior cannot successfully fake a psychiatric problem in order to avoid military service. Even those individuals with a history of psychiatric problems often have difficulty convincing draft examiners that the problems are severe enough to merit exemption. In short, the Soviet draft commissariat has considerably more data available on which it can determine the conscript's fitness for service than do most armies of the West.

Finally, the Soviets reduce psychiatric exemptions from military service by the simple practice of distinguishing between those individuals able to serve in combat units and noncombat units, respectively. In addition, based on the conscript's record and performance in premilitary training, some effort is made to select those who may be better fit for more complex and technical military assignments. These individuals also receive more extensive psychiatric screening, especially for such assignments as police units, missile units, and submarines. The Soviets seem to have come around to the idea that military manpower can be conserved by conscripting individuals with physical or even minor psychiatric problems for noncombat duties. The Soviets also maintain a large number of construction battalions to which almost anyone who meets even minimal standards can be assigned.

For the Soviets, military service goes quite beyond combat service. Because the state is seen as a mechanism for educating the young and disciplining them to the habits of obedience which a totalitarian regime requires, the Soviets view military service as an obligation that all citizens must observe. They are, then, quite prepared to find a place for almost everyone in the military even if this takes a little juggling; in general, they succeed in doing so. American intelligence estimates suggest that 92 percent of all conscripts called to military service eventually serve.[3] Many of those exempted are sent to reserve assignments. No doubt, much of this success is due to the Soviet view that psychiatrists are not allowed to interfere with the normal selection process to any great extent. The Soviets feel that too great a role for the military psychiatrist would probably result, as in the Western experience, in too great a rate of exemption from military service for psychiatric reasons.

Soviet Combat Medical Doctrine

Present Soviet combat medical doctrine was shaped by the experiences of World War I and II where the medical structure had to deal with enormous casualties. In the first six months of World War II, the Soviets lost 2.4 million men killed and wounded. They never had the capacity to treat this great number of mass casualties in an effective way. They have drawn three lessons from their experience, all of which remain central to their medical combat doctrine today.

The first lesson is that a medical system must be designed to handle the tremendous numbers of casualties engendered by war. The Soviets believe that the stress of war will make itself felt most clearly on the number of physical casualties which will be incurred and which can be saved through medical treatment. As in World War II, the Soviet medical corps neither intends nor is designed to treat psychiatric casualties seriously. Such casualties will be relegated to the area of small psychiatry and dealt with by political officers or within normal command channels. The Soviets expect to endure great numbers of physical casualties, especially if the war is fought (as they expect it to be) within a nuclear context. The emphasis on dealing with large numbers of casualties was characteristic of Soviet medical doctrine in World War II but has received renewed emphasis since 1967 when changes in Soviet battle doctrine forced them to examine seriously the impact of nuclear weapons on casualty rates.

A second lesson also emerged during World War II. The Soviets have completely integrated the entire civilian public health system into the military medical structure, so that the most serious casualties can be expected to be treated at front, army or district level hospitals. In World War II, the distinction between military and civilian hospitals and personnel was almost functionally nonexistent. Since the war, the Soviets have worked to almost totally eliminate the distinction. They have no intention of going to war without first mobilizing the entire civilian medical establishment and conscripting between 8,000 and 10,000 doctors for military service. The integration of military and civilian medical facilities, in an effort to mobilize the whole nation for war, is a major characteristic of the combat medical structure of the Soviet Army.

Finally, the third lesson is to evacuate casualties to rear areas for treatment rather than treat them at the front. Defense Intelligence Agency studies on Soviet combat medical treatment reveal that the emphasis is on treating the soldier in the unit only to the extent needed to keep him alive so that he can be evacuated to the rear rather than holding him at regiment or battalion and reintegrating him into his unit.[4] One reason for this practice is that the Soviets do not use a unit replacement system as do some of the Western armies. No real attempt is made to return wounded soldiers to their original units. During World War II, the Soviets copied the American system of individual replacement, thus supplanting the old regimental system characteristic of the armies of the czars and used in World War I and in the war against Finland. This reduced the traditional value of unit replacements which was a major distinguishing characteristic of European armies. It also affected the operation of the medical service system as it did in the American Army.

Like the Americans, the Soviets replace individuals rather than units. In World War II recovered wounded in the American Army did not normally return to their units but were sent to replacement depots (not to be confused with the replacement battalions of the German Army) where they were individually sent to various units as the need arose. However, the Soviets have made one important change in this practice. Soviet combat doctrine requires that units be fought down to 30 to 40 percent strength before being replaced. Rather than refilling a unit with individual replacements, the Soviets plan to commit another unit to battle in its place, linking the replaced unit with the replacing unit, passing command to the new unit, and continuing the assault. This means that a unit's membership and even command structure keep changing as the battle rages. Hence, the Soviets intend to evacuate their wounded and have them recover at army, front, or district hospitals where they will then be reassembled at replacement depots. At these depots whole new units will be formed and then thrown into battle so that there is no real possibility that Soviet soldiers will be returned to their original units. In fact, during World War II wounded soldiers were not allowed to return to their original units as a matter of policy, although in some cases recovering wounded left the replacement depots and tried to make their way back to their comrades.[5]

These three elements—emphasis on mass casualty treatment, integration of civilian and military medical structures, and evacuation of casualties to rear areas for treatment—are the major characteristics of the Soviet military medical system today. Medical treatment doctrine is essentially the same today as it was in World War II. After the war, the Soviets studied every aspect of the conflict in great detail, and their experience has profoundly affected the form and function of their medical service corps. The emphasis is on providing minimal medical treatment at each stage of the evacuation process, treating the casualty only to the extent needed to preserve his life and prepare him for the next move to the rear. Not much thought is given to stopping the flow of wounded to the rear and treating them at the battlefront so that they can be returned to their unit, at least not at the lower fighting echelons. The goal is to get the wounded to the rear as quickly as possible. New units are assembled and reconstructed from the recovering wounded in the replacement depots.

Soviet historical experience has been reinforced by modern developments, namely, the likelihood of fighting on a nuclear battlefield. It has been reinforced as well by the Soviet belief that the next major war will generate tremendous numbers of casualties as a result of chemical and biological agents. Thus, the Soviet medical corps is configured first and foremost to deal with mass casualties by getting them out of the way and not allowing them to hinder the ability of Soviet units to continue the offensive. This, in turn, is further supported by Soviet doctrine which requires a high tempo of battle in a continuous offensive to break the will of the enemy. Since the Soviets also believe that a war in the West will be a relatively short war, perhaps lasting no more than ninety days, they hope to be able to gain victory quickly by getting the most out of their troops over a short period of time. There will be plenty of time to treat the wounded and save what can be saved after their combat forces have defeated the enemy.

The Soviets do not seem to worry very much about the priority of medical treatment as a factor in maintaining combat effectiveness. Because they expect to fight a short, though very intense, war, they do not see the need for long-term medical treatment systems, especially when such systems might hinder the tempo of battle. One can obtain some idea of this doctrine in practice by understanding the Soviet doctrine of self-help for the soldier. This doctrine, openly taught to the troops, requires that the soldier be able to treat his own wounds or that of his comrades. This idea is important because the Soviet soldier is told that he may have to be left behind on the battlefield and may not receive any medical treatment at all, for the larger force will have to continue the advance. This view is radically different from that of the West where the soldier is continually assured that he will be well cared for if wounded and will never be abandoned. For the Western armies, this assurance is necessary to the soldier's morale and fighting ability. The Soviets, by contrast, emphasize that, whereas the treatment of the wounded is important, it is secondary to enabling the unit to continue the attack.

With the relatively low priority the Soviets place on treating the wounded as opposed to evacuating them, it is understandable that medical supplies are given the lowest priority in the logistics train.[6]

Unlike Western armies, few organic vehicles in the division are dedicated to medical evacuation, and almost none (as in the case of the Israeli Army) are dedicated to providing medical treatment. Although the Soviets are making some efforts to use helicopters in a medical evacuation role, these efforts are minimal and conditioned by the Soviet belief that the unarmed helicopter will be extremely vulnerable to hostile fire in a modern war. Accordingly, evacuation of the wounded to regimental and division collection points will be carried out not by organic vehicles dedicated to the task, but by empty supply carriers. Trucks and APCs will move to the front delivering POL and ammunition. On the way back to the rear resupply points, they will stop at regimental and divisional clearing stations to pick up the wounded and remove those tagged for evacuation. These factors—the emphasis on self-help and the possibility of being left alone, the absence of organic medical evacuation transport vehicles, and the low priority given to medical supplies in the logistics chain—suggest that the Soviets are not going to spend a great deal of time and effort treating casualties at the lower combat echelons. They will try to evacuate who they can to the rear as the tempo of battle permits. The major exception to this rule seems to be in the treatment of psychiatric casualties.

The lack of concern given to the treatment as opposed to the evacuation of casualties is reflected in the medical treatment structure. Soviet units have medical stations at company, battalion, regiment, and division level organized in pretty much the same fashion as in Western armies. However, in training military medical personnel, the emphasis is placed on their role in conducting the administrative task of moving casualties to the rear far more than on treating them at the front. At regiment and division, the chief medical officer functions almost entirely in an administrative rather than a medical capacity. It is only above division, at army or front level, that the wounded soldier receives any serious medical treatment. All other medical stations are seen essentially as through-put stations rather than as treatment stations.

What is the potential impact of Soviet medical evacuation policies on psychiatric casualties? It must be remembered that the Soviets intend to use the same diagnostic and screening mechanisms to deal with psychiatric casualties that they used in World War II. That means that a wide range of behavioral problems, which the West will treat as true neuropsychiatric problems, will be treated as cowardice, lack of motivation, lack of will, improper training, or defective character by the Soviets. Accordingly, large numbers of neuropsychiatric casualties (by Western standards) will not be allowed in the medical evacuation chain at all, but will be handled in administrative or command channels by the unit commanders or the political officers. In the modern Soviet Army, a political officer is assigned to every company, whereas in World War II, one was assigned to each battalion. They, therefore, have a much smaller number of personnel to deal with. One can reasonably expect the screening of psychiatric casualties to be somewhat more thorough than it was in World War II or than it can be expected to be in Western armies. Soviet medical and administrative personnel will likely refuse to recognize as legitimate any behavioral problem without an identifiable physical cause. To be sure, the truly psychotic will be evacuated in the medical chain. But the use of harsh diagnostic definitions of psychiatric damage should go a long way in keeping neuropsychiatric cases out of the medical evacuation chain as they did in World War II. For the most part, Soviet psychiatric casualties will be detained and treated in command channels or allowed to build up at the various medical clearing points where they receive the lowest priority for evacuation.

True neuropsychiatric casualties will be shunted into the normal medical evacuation chain and moved to the rear. Those soldiers who manifest concussion, contusion, or any other physiological problem associated with mental disturbance, will be moved to at least division level and, in many cases, further rearward. They will be given a period at the army level hospital of about two weeks to recover while in a neuropsychiatric ward. If they recover, they will then be assigned to a replacement depot for further utilization. Our knowledge of battleshock treatment in the West suggests that this practice may result in a greater number of deep neurosis casualties who might otherwise be turned around quickly. Once moved to the rear, secondary gain sets in and shock may deepen, so that the soldier may require a much longer time to recover. On the other hand, this may be balanced by the fact that if the Soviets can convince the patient that his problem is basically physiological in origin, once the physical aspects of the problem are handled, recovery may be fairly rapid.

If Western models are correct, between 30 and 40 percent of soldiers exposed to battle in a modern war can be expected to suffer a neuropsychiatric problem. The Soviet models offer different estimates. In their research, in which they calculate the shock effect of battle by using examples of shock effects found in natural disasters such as earthquakes, natural gas explosions, and large fires, Soviet military psychiatrists suggest that even in a nuclear battle zone they do not expect any more than 10 percent of the casualties to result from genuine neuropsychiatric reasons.[7] With no way of treating neuropsychiatric casualties in lower echelon holding areas on the grounds that casualties without physiological symptoms are not legitimately psychiatric at all, the Soviet medical support system may find itself greatly overburdened with neuropsychiatric casualties. Yet, if their filtration systems, namely, the command channels, political officers, and harsh clinical diagnostic definitions of what constitutes a mental casualty operate as effectively as they did in World War II, then the number of psychiatric casualties evacuated back to division may well be lower than that in Western armies.

The propensity to evacuate soldiers to the rear for medical treatment seems to have led the Soviets to use drug therapies at the lower levels of the medical treatment system to stabilize shock casualties and then move them to the rear. No one can reasonably foresee to what extent this will lead to misdiagnosis so that they may end up placing neuropsychiatric patients in the medical chain that otherwise could be treated much more rapidly and effectively at the front. The emphasis on drug therapies to counter the physiological effects that are expected to result from nuclear shock and battle stress may create serious problems for the medical service by evacuating casualties that simply should not have been evacuated.

These circumstances raise some questions about the quality of medical personnel who will conduct the diagnostic screening of psychiatric casualties. In general, the ability of military medical personnel to recognize genuine neuropsychiatric casualties is weak because of their emphasis on physiology. These personnel—sanitors, feldshers, and even regimental surgeons—may not be very well trained in the practical problems of recognizing and diagnosing neuropsychiatric casualties. This could result, first, in soldiers with a psychiatric syndrome that could be managed by lower level medical personnel being turned over to political officers and unit commanders without first receiving needed treatment. Second, it could result in the incorrect diagnosis and screening of large numbers of psychiatric casualties who would be evacuated rather than treated at the lower echelon levels. Soviet medical service generally deals with only the most severe neuropsychiatric symptomatologies, and in practice, such cases are handled through command or political channels. Only those symptomatologies accompanied by organic disruption can be adequately treated within the medical system. This suggests that soldiers with psychiatric problems unaccompanied by physical damage may easily be misdiagnosed, in which case they may be needlessly evacuated or forcibly returned to battle. The quality of medical training given to Soviet military medical personnel responsible for psychiatric cases is a real problem indeed. Even Western armies, for example, the Israeli Defense Force (IDF), share this problem. Although the IDF generally provides excellent doctors, psychiatrists, and psychologists in its field units, during the 1982 war in Lebanon, perhaps as many as half of the IDF's psychiatric casualty evacuations were misdiagnosed and needlessly evacuated to the rear.

The Soviets would apparently rather evacuate the normal physically damaged casualties than treat them at the front. One of their priorities is to stabilize and evacuate patients in biological shock. Those soldiers who suffer psychological reactions to physical damage are evacuated and treated as any other physical casualty. Those with psychiatric symptoms but no evidence of physical damage are either ignored, kept in local holding areas, or turned over to commanders and political officers.

Once a casualty reaches division, he is reexamined and a determination is made as to whether to retain him at the division hospital or move him further to the rear. Regardless of the level chosen, after two or three weeks special police units make regular rounds of military hospitals and treatment sites, selecting those soldiers who have sufficiently recovered from their wounds and sending them to replacement depots where they are assigned to new units and recommitted to battle. However else the Soviets handle the problem of evacuation of psychiatric casualties, they intend to make the doctrine of expectancy operate whether at the lower levels, where the soldier is turned over to the political officer or the unit commander, or at the higher levels, where the soldier is eventually sent to a replacement depot. The point is to convince the soldier that a psychiatric disturbance is not in itself a legitimate cause for escaping one's military responsibilities. Even genuine psychiatric casualties are expected to return to the fight. If they are treated at the lower level, they may return within a matter of hours and certainly days. Even if evacuated to division, they usually do not spend more than four to six weeks during which time a determination is made as to whether to return him to the fighting units or to discharge him as a permanent casualty into the public health system. Those who refuse to return are simply forced to return.

PSYCHIATRIC CASUALTY SERVICING STRUCTURE

At front level the Soviet Army maintains a complete psychiatric hospital with a director for psychiatric care and a special section for dealing with neuropsychiatric casualties. In addition, every military district has its own district hospital in which all medical specialties are available, including psychiatric care. The staff of the district hospital includes three or four neurologists and about the same number of psychiatrists. The Leningrad Military District Hospital, for example, has five neurologists and four psychiatrists on its staff, who care for inpatients, and perhaps two additional doctors, who care for military outpatients. The focus at both the front and district hospital is on neurology. In general, the military considers neurologists more valuable than psychiatrists because they can diagnose and treat the physical causes of brain disorders. The Soviets believe that the neurologist is more likely than the psychiatrist to look for physical damage as the cause of behavior.

The army level provides a small psychiatric ward that can accommodate up to forty beds. By and large, the psychiatric patient remains at army level for two weeks while undergoing treatment for minor psychiatric problems, three weeks if his problem is more serious, and no longer than six weeks if he has a truly serious problem. At the end of six weeks the patient is either sent to a replacement depot or turned over to the civilian psychiatric establishment for further treatment. A discharge is normally accompanied by the assessment that the soldier can no longer be of any functional military use even in noncombat assignments.

The division level has the normal complement of battle surgeons and doctors, but usually no psychiatrists or psychiatric wards. The division is seen as a combat fighting unit and is staffed mostly with medical surgical personnel who can deal with the common casualties of war. The Soviet Army has no equivalent of the Western army's division level psychiatrist. Nor is there a support staff of psychologists, social workers, or counselors which is so commonplace in Western armies, particularly in the Israeli and American armies. The problems which this staff usually handles are, in the Soviet Army, dealt with by the unit commander, his executive officer, or the political officer. At the division level the political officer has a small staff of four to five persons who are given more important tasks than dealing with psychiatric casualties.

The regimental level provides the normal medical staff comprised of a regimental surgeon and, sometimes, a neurologist but, again, there are no psychiatrists or psychologists. The problems of small psychiatry that surface there are dealt with by the unit commander or the political officer. The same is true at battalion level except that there is no doctor present. Medical treatment at battalion is handled by the battalion feldsher. As regards psychiatric casualties, the role of medical personnel below division is to separate the serious neuropsychiatric cases from the less serious ones. As in World War II, soldiers who are psychotic or have psychiatric symptoms that are easily attributable to a physical cause are evacuated to the next level where they are reexamined, treated and held for a few days, or shipped further to the rear, depending on the severity of the problem. Minor cases are turned over to command channels or the political officer and are handled on a "motivational basis." The first level at which a genuine neuropsychiatric casualty can be treated seriously is at army level. In the main, however, most instances of psychiatric disability are treated functionally at the lower level by short periods of rest and returned to the line.

The training of medics, feldshers, and even doctors in psychiatric triage is almost nonexistent, and whatever exists is far inferior to Western training. The prevailing notion is that too thorough a training of lower echelon medical personnel in psychiatric triage might result in an increase in psychiatric casualties as severe diagnostic definitions are eroded. There are no psychiatric assistants, as found in the American and Israeli armies, to help deal with psychiatric casualties. Although independent medical detachments have been set up under the authority of the medical department of the chief of the army front in order to help the divisions with medical problems, none of these special teams deals with psychiatric problems. For the most part they are nuclear, biological, and chemical teams, special surgical detachments, and even special equipment units that include specialists to handle problems caused by extreme weather environments. There are no special psychiatric teams similar to those used by the American Army in Vietnam or by the Israelis. In the Soviet medical structure up to army level, there are no organic staffs to deal with truly neuropsychiatric cases as a special problem area. Nor are there any attached medical facilities that can be pressed into action. Although there is a small neuropsychiatric ward at the army level hospital, and an even larger ward at the front level hospital, they are not usually staffed by psychiatrists. Most of the psychiatric work is done by neurologists.

Conversations with Soviet psychiatrists and battle surgeons reveal that the Soviet military is acutely aware that the presence of certain kinds of physicians within easy access of the troops tends to cause the troops to use the physicians' medical specialty as a way of avoiding duty or battle. Therefore, the Soviets do not position psychiatrists in their combat units and do not offer psychological services to the soldier at any level. In peacetime or in war, soldiers with problems cannot go to drug, alcohol, or family counselors; such facilities commonly exist only in Western armies. Soviet soldiers with problems are required to work them out by themselves or with the help of friends. As a rule, these problems come to the attention of the political officer or the unit commander only if they cause disruption in the expected behavior of the soldier. They are approached as disciplinary problems within the normal chain of command, and only rarely are they referred to medical personnel.

The political officer is a unique resource in the Soviet Army. Originally instituted to ensure the political loyalty of military commanders, the political officer has long since acquired more relevant functions. Only the Soviet Army has an officer and small staff within combat units who are directly responsible for ensuring the soldier's morale, motivation, and fighting spirit. In this sense, the political officer is an important adjunct to the commander. The Soviet commissar, although often denigrated in Western military literature, was often held in high esteem by soldiers in World War II. Combat histories of the Soviet Army show that the political officer was often the most motivated soldier in the unit and the most talented. Although many political hacks served as political officers, by and large this changed after the war. The Political Academy, which was founded prior to World War II, has been upgraded considerably, and most of the political officers today are college graduates. In addition, most have taken courses in psychology, if not psychiatry, to aid them in their primary function of maintaining morale and motivation. During World War II, the political officer was found only at battalion level or above. Today he is at company level as well and, at some point in the future, it is likely he will also be assigned to platoons.

Nicknamed the priest by the soldiers, the political officer is not usually sought out by the troops as a confidant and does not act as a counselor in the Western sense of the word. But he is charged with knowing what is going on among the troops in a unit, and, in practice, little escapes his attention. He is quite likely to seek out the problem soldier if only to remind him of his responsibilities. In this sense, he can function as the first line of defense in dealing with psychological problems. Again, however, the political officer approaches these problems as a member of the command staff and not as a medical practitioner. However, his personal participation in battle and his presence on the front line greatly increase his stature and authority in dealing with psychiatric problems. According to Soviet psychiatrists, these conditions often make him more effective than trained psychiatrists.

There are frequent behavioral problems among the soldiery, including very high rates of assaults on sergeants and even officers by common soldiers. The caste system within Soviet military units undoubtedly produces considerable stress. Soldiers are usually cooped up on their military bases, subject to harsh discipline, live in cramped quarters, are subject to the wrath of exploitative sergeants, and are given poor and monotonous diets. Even when they are granted a pass, it is usually not for overnight. When he is allowed off base, his sojourns are carefully controlled, and usually an officer or sergeant is present. There are few diversions and even fewer ways to relieve stress. Access to women is almost nonexistent, and there is a considerable amount of alcohol consumption in the Soviet military, although the amount of drinking in the military is probably less than that found in the society at large. Military life produces much greater stress for the Soviet soldier than for his Western counterpart, particularly the American soldier who would consider Soviet military life the equivalent of being in a prison. This stress frequently boils over into assaults on NCOs, and even officers, and leads to high rates of suicide.

When Soviet soldiers were asked, "Did you ever hear stories about people committing suicide in other units," 84.1 percent of the survey respondents indicated that they had heard such reports while in military service. At least 48.7 percent of the respondents reported that someone in their unit had attempted to commit suicide.[8] This rate of suicide attempts must be interpreted in light of the fact that many suicide attempts are really attempts to get a release from military service. From almost any perspective, however, it is apparent that the harshness of Soviet military life tends to produce psychiatric problems which in the Western army would require attention from either a psychiatrist, psychologist or, at least, counselor.

The soldier who is suffering from a psychiatric problem or who tries to commit suicide is almost always sent to prison. However, he may be held in jail for only a short time until a team of psychiatrists from the army or front level hospital can interview him and diagnose his problem. Even this type of examination requires a request from his commanding officer who, in making such a request, is admitting that he cannot handle the situation. As such, sending for a psychiatrist to examine a problem soldier is likely to occur only after the commander and the political officer have made repeated attempts to manage by themselves. If an examination reveals that the problem is essentially behavioral rather than physiological, the soldier is usually turned back to his commander for punishment or retained in prison. If, on the other hand, the soldier is truly mentally ill, he is usually sent back to a rear area military hospital for treatment. If his problem can be cured, or at least dealt with, he is then returned to his unit to complete his military service. The time spent in the hospital is often not counted against his military enlistment; in short, it is "bad time" that must be made up.

The soldier with a diagnosis of a serious psychiatric problem that cannot be treated by the military medical system is turned over to the public health system and discharged from the service. The rate of discharge for psychiatric problems in peacetime is very low, for the Soviet authorities do not want to set a precedent. Therefore, soldiers with psychiatric problems not originating in organic causes are dealt with very severely, and every effort is made to keep them in military service even if they cannot be useful members. In the Soviet view, it is more important for other soldiers to know that psychiatric debilitation cannot be rewarded with release from military service.

PSYCHIATRIC TREATMENT

In their treatment of psychiatric patients the Soviets have historically stressed therapies based in biological theory. This practice is based on the assumption that all behavior, including aberrant behavior, is traceable to organic disruption of brain functions. This approach has been characteristic of Russian psychiatry since before the turn of the century, and it is equally characteristic of Soviet military psychiatry today. With the partial rehabilitation of Soviet psychology as a separate discipline after the mid–1960s, there has been a rise in what the Soviets generically term "socio-rehabilitative therapies." By 1981, Soviet textbooks on the subject were calling each approach—the socio-rehabilitative and the biological—"equally important." Nonetheless, the medical doctor, usually a neurologist or a psychiatrist, and not the psychologist, remains the predominant figure and generally oversees treatment. The biological approach is still dominant, and the mental hospitals are only rarely staffed by psychologists or other mental therapists. In those few situations where psychologists are allowed to conduct therapy, they are often formally informed that the law requires that a medical doctor, often a neurologist, be present or oversee treatment. Nonbiological therapies are regarded with suspicion in the psychiatric establishment.

Basic biological therapies have been evident in Soviet military psychiatry at least since 1905 and have their parallel in the West. Among the more common therapies are somatic, physical, active, narcotic sleep, insulin comatose, medical convulsive, and electroconvulsive therapies. With the rise of what the Soviets call the "pharmacological era of psychiatry," which they date from French research into psychotropic drugs in the 1950s, many of these basic biological shock therapies have been replaced by drug-based therapies. Soviet psychiatrists are apparently enthusiastic about drug intervention therapies and suggest that the use of psychopharmacological agents

has spread the boundaries of therapeutic action, changed the appearance of psychiatric hospitals and revealed new possibilities for social labor readaptation with the return of patients to society and labor activity. Because of the simplicity of use, speed and impact on the psychological disorders and the comparative safety of these substances, the volume of psychiatric aid has considerably increased and extended the possibilities of extra-hospital treatment.[9]

By the early 1970s, the drug revolution in the Soviet Union had taken full hold, and it now has a major role in psychiatry. For a list of major drugs used in Soviet psychiatric practice, along with the conditions for which they are prescribed, see Table 5.

Despite the increase in the use of drug-related therapeutic techniques, control over therapies for treating combat shock or other mental problems in the military still resides with psychiatrists and neurologists. The concept of drug therapy has actually strengthened the idea of the organic origin of mental aberration, and drugs seem an excellent therapy to psychiatrists inasmuch as they work directly on the physiological functions of the brain. Thus, "drugs address the brain and have points of application in the specific material structure of the brain and produce complex neurotrophic effects."[10]

With regard to the state of Soviet psychotherapy, it still has the suspicious reputation it acquired under Stalinism. Psychotherapy in the Soviet lexicon is defined as "a complex and therapeutic action with the aid of the mental substances on the patient's psyche and through it to the entire organism for the purpose of eliminating morbid symptoms and changing the relation of the organism to itself and to its state and to its environment."[11] This definition is vague and unspecific as to function, as are the therapies that have arisen from it. Among psychotherapeutic treatments are rational psychotherapy, autosuggestion, suggestion in a state of wakefulness, autogenic training, hypnosis or hypnotherapy, and narcopsychotherapy. In psychotherapy, the use of psychotropic

Table 5
Drugs Used by Soviet Military Psychiatrists in Treatment of Neurosis and Psychosis

For Psychosis
  Antipsychotics
    Sedatives: (aminazine, propazin, levopromazine, chlorprotixine, reserpine, leponex)
    Selectives: (triftazin, meterazine, haloperidol, carbidin, pimozide)
    Generals: (mazheptyl, trisedyl)
    Mood elevators: (thyoridazine, perphenazine, frenolon, fluorophenazine, fluspiridine, pimozide, eglonyl)
  Antidepressants
    Sedatives: (amitriptylene, surmontyl, azaphine, fluoracisin, prothiaden, oxylidine, pyrazidol)
    Thymoanaleptics: (imizine, pertofran, anafranil, nortriptyline)
    Stimulants: (iprazide, nuredal, benazide, transamine, nitrazepam)

For Reactive States/Neurosis
  Tranquilizers
    Sedatives: (meprobamate, amizyl, chlordiazepoxide, oxazepam, nitrazepam, phenazepam, mebicar)
  Stimulators
    Minor mood elevators: (trioxazin, diazepam, medazepam)
    Psychostimulants: (pervitin, meridil, piridrol, syndocarb, centrophinoxine, pyriditol)

Source: G. Avrutskiy and A. A. Neduva, *Treatment of the Mentally Ill* (Moscow: Meditsina, 1981), p. 56.

drugs is an essential component of the complex therapeutic action, and the value of such drugs is seen to lie basically in their ability to treat the organic causes of brain disfunction. Thus, Soviet psychologists have made the appropriate bow in the direction of the dominant psychiatrists and their organic orientation toward psychiatric illness.

The Soviets have engaged in clinical psychotherapy only since the mid-1970s, and, as a result, many of their treatment therapies have still not attained general acceptance. They have also had some difficulty in establishing the connection between therapies and success rates because they lack sufficient data bases to make statistical comparisons. Psychotherapy as practiced by Soviet psychologists is still carefully controlled, for a public law guiding the use of psychotherapies is still in effect. This law, first promulgated by the People's Commissariat of Public Health, requires that psychotherapy must be conducted at all times in the presence of a psychiatrist or a physician. This decree was originally issued in 1926 and in Soviet textbooks remains the main guideline for the use of psychotherapy in clinical situations.

Soviet psychiatry, with its biological emphasis, seems to be moving toward predicting and thus preventing improper social behavior. Just as physical medicine can have a preventive form so, too, can a physiologically based psychiatry. As the Soviets expand their concerns of psychology to include work behavior and rehabilitation for aberrant behavior, the use of preventive psychiatry is expected to grow. A totalitarian state can always find use for a diagnostic science that can identify social deviants before they act out their deviance. One indication of this trend toward preventive psychiatry can be seen in the establishment of psychoprisons staffed by both psychiatrists and psychologists.

Soviet psychiatrists rely heavily on drug therapies to deal with problems resulting from battle stress as well as other trauma. The Soviets maintain that there is nothing unique about battle per se which produces unique reactions to stress. Much of Soviet research on the subject tends to reinforce the belief that many symptoms of stress encountered on the battlefield can be found as readily in civilian disaster occurrences, such as plane crashes, large fires, tornadoes, and earthquakes. Therefore, the treatments offered to soldiers suffering from combat psychosis and civilians suffering from psychosis induced by other factors are much the same.

In their treatment of stress, the Soviets have continuously made use of folk and herb medicines, and a number of these compounds are still in some use today including such natural tranquilizers and stimulants as valeriana and pantacrene. Others, such as chloryl hydrate and cardiac bromide, are still used widely, as are calcium and magnesium IVs. Soviet psychiatrists believe these natural compounds have some advantages over alternative chemical compounds. They can generally be taken orally in droplet form; they do not overstimulate the system; they are not usually followed by exhaustion; and they are more easily absorbed by the body than are most synthetic compounds. On the battlefield, sanitors and feldshers carry medical kits that contain pills, liquids, and even injections of these natural compounds along with the basic drugs for treating stress reactions. Despite their popularity, the basic object of Soviet military treatments for stress reactions is to develop synthetic drugs. Psychopharmacology is rapidly coming of age in the Soviet Union, and its developments tend to parallel those in the West.

The Soviets are trying to adopt essentially the same diagnostic criteria used in the West for treating syndromes specifically related to battle stress. As noted earlier, the Ministry of Health has enforced the use of ICD–9 on the public health system in an effort to standardize diagnostic criteria. In general, the Soviets use many of the same major diagnostic categories for defining battleshock-related problems as they use in dealing with shock reactions resulting from other causes. In handling battleshock reactions, Soviet military psychiatry uses diagnostic categories that emphasize reactive states. They further subcategorize reactive states into acute shock reactions, depressive reactions, and reactive delirious psychosis. Other diagnostic categories related to battleshock include neurosis, neurasthenia, hysterical neurosis, and hysterical psychosis. A diagnostic category that is not used very much in the West but that has a long history of use in the Soviet military addresses those symptomatic psychoses resulting from infectious diseases. A relatively complete list of diagnostic categories, including those frequently used in the West that are not used by Soviet psychiatrists, is presented in Tables 6 and 7. It is interesting to examine how the Soviets functionally define these diagnostic categories and what specific treatments are recommended for each.

Table 6
Symptom Indicators Used by Soviet Military Psychiatrists to Diagnose Battle Neurosis and Psychosis

For Neurosis	For Psychosis
Irritability	Depression
Fatigue	Melancholia
Nervousness	Abulia
Insomnia	Apathy
Anxiety	Stupor
Phobia	Agitation
Low suppressed mood	Compulsion
Hypochondria	Delusion
Iatrogenia	Hallucination
Obsession	Denial of disease
	Depersonalization
	Extreme anxiety

Table 7
Common Terms Used in Western Military Psychiatry That Are Not Used by Soviet Military Psychiatrists

Post-traumatic stress disorder
Anxiety disorder
Battleshock syndrome
Neurotic depression

Soviet military psychiatry maintains that reactive states are caused by short-term traumatic impacts on the soldier. For the Soviets trauma refers exclusively to physical injury, not, as in the United States, to the nonphysical impact of psychological reactions. The onset of a reactive state is very rapid and, therefore, is clearly distinguished from the effects of long-term battle fatigue. Reactive states can set in within hours or even minutes of exposure to trauma. In the Soviet view, psychotic reactions are directly related to the nature and intensity of the traumatic event and are not a mechanism for triggering deeper psychological problems. In addition, the reversibility of a psychotic reaction is in direct proportion to the degree and impact of the initial trauma, a notion that fits very well with the traditional idea that trauma acts primarily to disrupt the physiology of the brain by disordering the conditioned reflexes of the second signal system.

The Soviets maintain that their view of trauma-induced psychosis as caused by a disruption of brain function is very realistic, and they define reactive states as having certain characteristics. The first characteristic of a reactive state is functionality: it is a functional response to stress which allows the soldier to escape from battle or to close off some horror he may have witnessed. Accordingly, the Soviets understand the problem of secondary gain. They understand that a soldier "gains" or profits from remaining in his reactive state, and, as way of approaching treatment, they make every effort to demonstrate to the soldier, either through traumatic therapy or threats of punishment, that this gain will not be tolerated. A second characteristic of reactive states is their reversibility and temporary nature, a view directly deducible from their assumption that the brain learns by conditioned response. The objective of treatment is to recondition the brain or shock it back into its normal pattern of operation. Once the trauma abates and the brain returns to working normally again, the reactive state should dissipate. In short, if brain patterns have been disordered by trauma, the removal of the trauma—or the infliction of stronger stimuli—ought to break the psychosis. There is simply no question of psychosis lingering in the absence of trauma in the sense that it results from deeper psychological problems which the trauma happened to bring to the surface. A third characteristic is the essentially nonpsychogenic nature of reactive states: that is, reactive states do not result from long-standing psychological problems. Instead, they are a specific and temporary response to traumatic conditions which the organism has suffered. The removal of the soldier from these conditions is often sufficient to reverse the syndrome.

As noted earlier, Soviet military psychiatrists clinically distinguish three types of affective battle reactions: acute affective shock, depressive psychogenic shock, and reactive delirious psychosis. In acute affective shock, the onset of the reactive state is very rapid and takes many forms, including paralysis, blindness, and surdomutism. Rarely will acute reactions produce a psychogenic stupor, but they will occur from time to time. In general, the Soviets place stupor in the category of depressive reactions. To treat acute reactive shock, the Soviets immediately isolate the individual from the traumatic event and move the patient out of the risk zone. They also try to insulate him from the rest of the members of his unit in order to prevent any contagion (although the contagion effect is denied any validity in Soviet psychiatric theory.) If necessary, the soldier is immobilized with restraints. Drugs are administered immediately to stabilize the patient. Frequent use of heavy impact doses, as much as 100 to 150 milligrams, are given by injection on the spot until the sedative effect takes hold. The drugs of choice to treat acute affective shock are phenazapen, phenazepam, ilenium, siduzin, and amitriptylene, all of which are strong tranquilizers. After the patient has been sedated, other tranquilizing doses are administered to sustain the sedated condition. These less powerful but sustaining compounds include aminazine, tisercin, and chlorprotixine. They are also administered in relatively high doses until the patient has recovered.

The Soviets find that the most common manifestation of reactive psychosis is what they call depressive reactions. Here they recommend an intense therapy utilizing amitriptylene, an antidepressant. Again the practice is to administer heavy initial doses to prevent a deepening of the depression. They distinguish between types of depression and prescribe different degrees of drug doses to deal with them. In general, however, a true psychotic depression is treated with high doses of ampriptylene, melipramine, and pyrazidol. Shallow depression seems to respond fairly well to high doses of azaphine.

Reactive delirious psychosis, a severe reactive depression accompanied by strong physiological symptoms, is referred to as a "tightened reactive state" by Soviet psychiatrists. It is characterized by such extreme symptoms as delirium of pursuit, auditory hallucinations, surdomutism, and a complete disassociation from reality. In treating this condition, the Soviets have made use of neuroleptics such as triftazin, perphenazine, and trisedyl. They recognize the validity of a number of psychotraumatizing situations encountered in battle. These situations can cause extreme psychomotor excita-

Soviet Battlefield Psychiatry

tion in the soldier which may last for several hours. The symptoms include sensory delirium, false perceptions, and strong affective fear. Soviet psychiatrists suggest that strong and immediate treatment be rendered to deal with these symptoms before the syndrome can gain a strong hold on the individual. Their experience suggests that the rapidity of treatment is fundamental to reversing the reaction. Reactive delirious psychosis is treated like cases of acute shock, and the therapy of choice is to administer strong neuroleptics with sedative effects. Some more commonly prescribed drugs used in these cases include aminazine, levopromazine, chlorphophysine, and tryphotizine, all given intramuscularly and in high doses.

In specific cases of extreme psychomotor excitation resulting from trauma, the use of aminazine and levopromazine at 25 to 50 milligrams a day by injection is recommended. Also used is a 2 percent solution of dimedrol, a 25 percent solution of magnesium sulphate, or a solution of barbamyl in combination with a 10 percent solution of glucanated calcium and 10 percent calcium chloride administered intravenously. In the treatment of hysterical stupor, the use of psychomotor stimulants is prescribed using syndocarb at 30 to 40 milligrams a day accompanied by a mild tranquilizer.

Soviet military psychiatrists stress that reactive psychosis is strongly associated with battle stress. They are indeed aware of other kinds of reactions to battleshock, but their primary emphasis seems to be on dealing with reactive psychosis and the reason is clear enough. If one takes the view that the soldier's behavior is totally a function of the organic operations of the brain and that any disruption of brain functions will produce physiological symptoms (and vice versa), then the focus on the strong physiological symptoms that accompany reactive psychosis is logical. For Soviet military psychiatrists, reactive psychosis has become a kind of "bottom line." It is here that the soldier will most commonly manifest the kinds of problems that will have the greatest effect on the combat unit. More importantly, reactive psychosis is accompanied by clear physiological disruptions and symptomatology which facilitate diagnosis by a psychiatrist rather than a battle surgeon. The Soviets, therefore, tend to emphasize reactive states in their treatment of battle stress. In reactive psychosis, the Soviet psychiatrist has the precise case for which he or she is best trained to deal, namely, a psychiatric disturbance caused by a physiological trauma that manifests itself in external symptoms which can be dealt with directly, usually through drug therapy, and which affect the organic operations of the brain. Understandably, then, Soviet military psychiatrists seem to concentrate on reactive psychosis as the most important form of neuropsychiatric breakdown that they will have to deal with in future wars.

Although Soviet military psychiatrists are quite capable of recognizing a wide range of other battleshock reactions, they apparently expend little effort on treating them. In the treatment of neurosis, for example, which they see as a consequence of fear and anxiety, Soviet psychiatrists are likely to regard this as a minor problem and to treat it with short-term tranquilizer therapy. Except when the neurosis is deep and debilitating, they will define the condition as appropriate to small psychiatry, to be handled appropriately outside medical channels. In treating neurosis, vegeostabilizers are used to break down the physiological disruptions in the organism which are the cause of fear and anxiety. Soviet psychiatrists take neurasthenia only slightly more seriously. This malady takes the form of weakness, exhaustion, reduction of mental and physical efficiency, transitions of mood, and inability to focus and process information. These symptoms are regarded as hypostenic as opposed to hyperstenic forms of neurasthenia. The major treatment recommended is tranquilizer therapy to break the organic reaction patterns (what the Soviets call vegetative autonomic nervous system patterns). The hyperstenic form (an interesting diagnosis in itself) is characterized by an extreme form of excitation. Once again, tranquilizing drugs are recommended, including meprobamate, emisile, ilenium, trapazine, and phenazecom. In its hypostenic form, neurasthenia is treated with antidepressant drugs and stimulants, including trioxazin, sougexin, and the psychostimulants syndocarb and sindophine. The Soviets emphasize that, as with other battle stress-related problems, the treatment of neurasthenia should begin as quickly as possible. They emphasize that the possibility of psychological dependence on drugs should also be monitored.

Soviet psychiatrists seem to have achieved some success in the treatment of asthenic states through the use of a new class of drugs called nootropes. This new class of drugs is believed to work basically by affecting the metabolism of the cells of the brain. Examples are iminalon and ancebol. Not much information about the efficacy of these drugs or their chemical composition is available, but one Soviet pharmacologist noted that they were invented in Japan as GABA derivatives and are, in fact, widely used in Europe where they are manufactured under license.

Soviet military psychiatrists also recognize three other categories of battleshock reactions: hysterical neurosis, hysteria, and psychasthenia. Hysterical neurosis is characterized by short-term, reversible, and psychogenically nonpsychotic disorders. Examples of this condition are temporary mutism, asthasia, abasia, hysterical fits, and weeping. The specific conditions that separate hysterical neurosis from reactive psychosis are unclear; one distinguishing factor seems to be the rapidity with which the patient responds to treatment. Thus, the initial treatments for dealing with hysterical neurosis are the traditional ones (used in World War I by almost all armies) of slapping or shaking the soldier, shouting, causing pain, immersion in cold water, or any other means of causing a shock to the patient in order to bring him out of his condition. More modern treatments follow if traditional means do not work. These treatments require the administration of drugs such as ilenium and phenazepam by injection.

Two other categories of battleshock are hysteria and psychasthenia. Hysteria is defined as affective instability expressed in behavior and is generally characterized by the same symptoms as hysterical neurosis, although not as deeply. The treatment of choice is either shock or tranquilizers. Pyschasthenia is characterized by an alarming overanxiousness and uncertainty about one's abilities and surroundings, usually accompanied by lowered moods. The use of psychostimulators is indicated in the treatment of this condition.

The Soviets have also identified a type of psychiatric disruption that is organically based and that seems almost absent from American literature. This is a type of psychiatric, often psychotic, reaction to poisoning or infectious disease. This condition is called exogenic symptomatic psychosis and, according to the Soviets, is based in the disrupted physiology of the patient. Soviet military psychiatrists identify five basic types of symptomatic psychosis: delirium, epileptic excitation, twilight states, confusion, and hallucinations. Because armies have historically suffered as many or more casualties from disease as from enemy fire, the focus on mental aberrations caused by disease processes probably has a long history in Soviet military medicine. Moreover, it is the kind of problem that would find a ready audience within Soviet psychiatry. Because organic patterns may be disrupted not only by battleshock but also by disease, fever, and viruses, the Soviet military psychiatrist is comfortable in dealing with the psychiatric effects of infectious diseases.

In reading Soviet military medical literature, one is struck by its emphasis on the treatment of mental disruptions caused by the external environment. The impact of such hostile climates of extreme heat and cold on the soldier's ability to maintain the mental strength to continue the battle has been closely studied. This research direction is only moderately evident in American military psychiatry, and, where it is, it is not reflected in the research of psychiatrists as much as in the work of battle surgeons. In the Soviet case, one again encounters the tendency to join the medical doctor and the psychiatrist at the point of common origin, where the physiological disruption of the brain produces behavioral aberrations.

7
Future Directions of Soviet Military Psychiatry

The future directions of Soviet psychiatric research and field applications will likely continue to focus on the "revolution in psychopharmacology," that is, on the use of drugs both to prevent and treat psychiatric illnesses resulting from combat stress. Soviet military psychiatry will not likely abandon its basic assumptions regarding patterned responses in the brain as the explanation of human behavior, if for no other reason than that they worked well during World War II. In the Soviet view, their applications of combat psychiatry have already proven themselves to be far superior to those of the West insofar as they were able to preserve their manpower base during the Great Patriotic War. They fully expect that these same assumptions will prove effective in the next war.

Psychology, as a separate discipline, is in a somewhat less certain and secure position. The development of psychology in the Soviet Union has moved relatively slowly since the mid–1960s and early 1970s. It has been forced to accommodate its research and findings to the predominantly biological view of the human psyche held by both the regime and the dominant psychiatric establishment. It is doubtful that a truly independent field of military psychology in the Soviet Union exists or that one will be allowed to develop. Although there is some evidence that Soviet psychologists are attempting to emulate the kinds of surveys and data bases that are now commonplace in the West, progress has been comparatively slow. Moreover, some psychologists believe that they should explore the Western view that human behavior is sometimes rooted in purely emotional factors for which no easily discernible physical cause can be found, but Soviet psychology is not secure enough to risk pursuing the possibility. For the last fifteen years, the resuscitated discipline of psychology has been directed into the area of engineering psychology where corellations can be made between performance and physiological characteristics. If and when Soviet psychology is allowed to move in the direction of Western research—and it is by no means certain that it will be allowed to do so—it will do so slowly and cautiously, and will take a very long time. Thus, the prognosis is that Soviet military psychology will remain considerably behind the West for at least the foreseeable future.

For at least the next decade, then, Soviet psychiatry and psychology will remain essentially as they have been for the last twenty years. Neither discipline will likely produce any truly revolutionary developments. It seems to be a characteristically Russian way of approaching things to proceed gradually, only slowly incorporating incremental changes. Yet, it must be said that, although Soviet psychiatry, especially in relation to its diagnosis and treatment of battle stress-related illnesses, proceeds fundamentally from premises that are regarded as highly questionable in the United States, in practice, their system seems to work fairly well in dealing with psychiatric casualties. No one can deny that in World War II the Soviets had a much lower rate of manpower loss due to psychiatric problems than did most allied armies, particularly the United States. Furthermore, the political structure reinforces the diagnostic categories and treatment mechanisms used by the Soviet military psychiatric establishment. Western armies used essentially the same diagnostic criteria and treatments during World War I.

Perhaps it is a truism that men will generally behave as they are expected to behave by the subculture that sets the standards and values of behavior. Or perhaps, as a corollary, the process involved in the evolution of symptomatic indicators of mental breakdown is not as confused as it might first appear. Men under stress seem often to exhibit the very symptoms spelled out in the diagnostic categories used by medical examiners to decide if a man is to be removed from stressful situations. Hence, if a severe case of the "war tremors" is sufficient to permit a soldier to escape battle, then it comes as no surprise to discover that soldiers tend to develop precisely this condition when the horrors of war increase. In the Soviet case, if reactive psychosis is what is required to obtain relief from battle, then Soviet soldiers will likely develop reactive psychosis. This means that the values of the military subculture may well play a much larger role in determining the combat reactions an army will eventually suffer once it is committed to battle. The harshness of treatment for certain kinds of combat reactions may in itself also affect the frequency of psychiatric breakdown. Certainly, the Soviets seem to believe this is the case and have designed their theory and practice of combat psychiatry accordingly.

There are two different types of systems for defining and dealing with psychiatric battle casualties. Each system can be distinguished from the other in terms of the rigidity of its diagnostic categories and the manner in which psychiatric patients are treated. In general, the systems used by both the Soviet Army and German Army in World War II were far stricter than those used by the U.S. Army in that war and the Israeli Army in the Lebanon war of 1982. It would appear that the more severe systems proved more effective than the lenient ones in reducing manpower loss to psychiatric casualties. By comparison, the Soviet and German armies in World War II suffered about the same psychiatric casualty loss rate of approximately 9 men per 1,000. In the case of the United States, the loss rate for ground forces was about 36 per 1,000. In the case of the Israelis in Lebanon, their psychiatric casualties, approximately 600, outnumbered the total dead by almost two times, and this in only a limited war lasting six days characterized by generally light combat.

Perhaps military psychiatry is no more removed from any other discipline that must put its theories into practice. When theory becomes institutionalized as structure and power, theoretical propositions and analytical categories risk becoming self-fulfilling prophecies. In the realm of things psychic, perhaps what ultimately matters most are the values and expectations that men have of themselves and their peers. These factors, more than any other, may have the most determining effect on the behavior of men under fire. The Soviets seem to think this is the case, and their military psychiatry will probably continue to reflect this view until events prove them wrong . . . or right.

Notes

1. ORIGINS OF SOVIET PSYCHIATRY AND PSYCHOLOGY

1. Neal Miller, Carl Pfallmann, and Harold Schlossberg, *Soviet Psychology* (Princeton, N. J.: Princeton University Press, 1961), p. 90.
2. Ibid., p. 91.
3. Ibid., p. 95.
4. Ibid., p. 93.
5. The figure of 22,000 was valid as of 1979. It was obtained in conversations with a former official of the Soviet Academy of Science, one of whose tasks was to keep a record of the membership roles.
6. Ruth Daniloff, "Softening the Strains of Soviet Life," *Psychology Today* (April 1984), p. 49.
7. Ibid., p. 50.
8. Interview with a former employee of the institute.
9. Estimate provided by analysts of the Foreign Science and Technology Center, Charlottesville, Virginia.
10. Ibid.
11. Ibid.

2. DEVELOPMENT OF SOVIET MILITARY PSYCHIATRY

1. R. L. Richards, "Mental and Nervous Disease in the Russo-Japanese War," *The Military Surgeon*, Vol. 26 (1910), p. 179.

2. Richard A. Gabriel, "Stress in Battle: Coping on the Spot," *Army Magazine* (December 1982), pp. 36–42. Further information was obtained in an interview with Dr. David Marlowe, chairman of the Department of Military Psychiatry, Army Institute of Research, Walter Reed Hospital, Washington, D.C.

3. Richards, "Mental and Nervous Disease," p. 180.

4. Ibid.

5. Ibid., p. 185.

6. Ibid., pp. 186–187.

7. Ibid., p. 185. Figures calculated from the gross data provided in the chart on p. 185.

8. My thanks to John Windhausen, professor of Russian History at St. Anselm College for his help in assembling information on the Russian famine.

9. Josef Brozek, "Fifty Years of Soviet Psychology: An Historical Perspective," *Soviet Psychology*, Vol. 3, No. 1 (Fall 1968), pp. 48–57.

10. Ibid., p. 52.

11. Ibid.

12. A number of Soviet psychiatrists interviewed for this project reported using these techniques in World War II. They also indicated that such techniques were presented in their medical school lectures as being derived from Russian battle experience in World War I.

13. This document was brought to my attention by a graduate of the Kirov Military Medical Academy. An academy professor helped do the research for the work. After two years of searching, this writer's best guess as to its location is in a medical library in East Germany.

14. T. R. Dupuy, *The Encyclopedia of Military History* (New York: Harper and Row, 1970), p. 1198.

15. Interview with Lieutenant Colonel Robert Glantz, U.S. Army War College, Carlisle Barracks, Pennsylvania, July 23, 1984.

16. Eli Ginsburg, *The Lost Divisions* (New York: Columbia University Press, 1959), p. 93.

17. Ibid., p. 35.

18. Glantz interview, July 23, 1984.

19. Ginsburg, *The Lost Divisions*, p. 61.
20. Ibid., p. 100.
21. Estimates provided by Professor David Marlowe and Colonel Mike Camp of the Department of Military Psychiatry at the Army Institute of Research at Walter Reed Hospital.

3. SOVIET COMBAT PSYCHIATRY IN WORLD WAR II

1. Interview with Colonel Robert Glantz of the Strategic Studies Institute of the U.S. Army War College as cited earlier in this work.
2. Walter S. Dunn, Jr., "People Policies In Combat," *Parameters*, Vol. 14, No. 1 (Spring 1984), pp. 49–59.
3. This information was supplied through interview with Soviet psychiatrists and battle surgeons who served in World War II.

4. MODERN SOVIET MILITARY PSYCHIATRIC THEORY

1. V. V. Shelyag, A. D. Glotochkin, and K. K. Platonov, eds., *Military Psychology: A Soviet View* (Moscow: Government Publishing House, 1972), Translated by U.S. Air Force, p. 7.
2. Ibid., p. 8.
3. I. M. Sechenev, *The Reflexes of the Brain* (Moscow: Government Publishing House, 1947), p. 176.
4. Ibid., pp. 176–177.
5. Leonid Pavlovich Grimak, *The Psychological Training of the Parachutist* (Moscow: Government Publishing House, 1971), Translated by the Defense Technical Information Center, p. 22.
6. Ibid., p. 26.
7. Ibid., p. 27.
8. Ibid., p. 31.
9. Shelyag et al., *Military Psychology*, p. 249.
10. Ibid.
11. Ibid., p. 250.
12. Ibid., p. 169.
13. Ibid., pp. 174–176.
14. Ibid., p. 175.
15. Grimak, *The Psychological Training of the Parachutist*, p. 55.
16. Ibid.

17. Ibid.
18. Ibid., p. 54.
19. Ibid.
20. Ibid., p. 168.
21. Shelyag et al., *Military Psychology*, p. 363.
22. Grimak, *The Psychological Training of the Parachutist*, p. 186.
23. Shelyag et al., *Military Psychology*, p. 211.
24. David Marlowe, "Cohesion, Anticipated Breakdown, and Endurance in Battle: Considerations for Severe and High Intensity Combat" (Washington, D.C.: Walter Reed Army Institute of Research, 1979), Draft Paper, pp. 2–3.
25. Shelyag et al., *Military Psychology*, p. 209.
26. Reuven Gal and Richard Gabriel, "Battlefield Heroism in the Israeli Defense Force," *International Social Science Review* (Autumn 1982), pp. 233–235.
27. Grimak, *The Psychological Training of the Parachutist*, p. 152.
28. Ibid., p. 153.

5. PREVENTING BATTLE STRESS

1. Christopher Donnelly, "The Soviet Attitude Toward Stress in Battle," paper circulated at the conference on the Soviet Fighting Man sponsored by the Canadian Army at Gagetown, New Brunswick, in January 1983, p. 17.
2. Leonid Pavlovich Grimak, *The Psychological Training of the Parachutist* (Moscow: Government Publishing House, 1971), Translated by the Defense Technical Information Center, p. 16.
3. Donnelly, "Soviet Attitude Toward Stress," p. 14.
4. Ibid., p. 15.
5. Richard A. Gabriel, *The Mind of the Soviet Fighting Man* (Westport, Conn.: Greenwood Press, 1984), p. 30 (Table 53).
6. Ibid.
7. Ibid. Table 52.
8. David Marlowe, "Cohesion, Anticipated Breakdown and Endurance in Battle: Considerations for Severe and High Intensity Combat" (Washington, D.C.: Walter Reed Army Institute for Research, 1979) Draft Paper, pp. 2–4.
9. Colonel A. Voropal, "The Medical Officer and Psychological Training," *Soviet Military Review* (November 1977), p. 28.

10. Gabriel, *The Mind of the Soviet Fighting Man*, p. 12 (Table 13).
11. Ibid. Table 14.
12. Donnelly, "Soviet Attitude Toward Stress," p. 3.
13. I am indebted to Stephen P. Dalziel of the Soviet Studies Research Center at Sandhurst, England, for his help in explaining the connection between these three factors and the development of Soviet combat tactics.
14. Donnelly, "Soviet Attitude Toward Stress," p. 18.
15. G. Avrutskiy and A. A. Neduva, *Treatment of the Mentally Ill* (Moscow: Government Publishing House [Meditsina], 1981, p. 3.
16. Ibid., p. 48.

6. SOVIET BATTLEFIELD PSYCHIATRY

1. See note 3 in Chapter 3 of this work.
2. Information about this study was provided by Soviet medical personnel now living in the West who took part in the study or had direct first-hand knowledge of its existence.
3. This figure is provided by Defense Intelligence Agency analysts who specialize in studying the personnel policies of the Soviet Army.
4. *Medical Support of the Soviet Ground Forces* (Washington, D.C.: Defense Intelligence Agency Report, March 1979), p. 8.
5. Walter S. Dunn, "People Policies in Combat," *Parameters*, Vol. 14, No. 1 (Spring 1984), pp. 49–50.
6. *Medical Support of the Soviet Ground Forces*, p. 4.
7. Estimate provided in interviews with Soviet military psychiatrists.
8. Richard A. Gabriel, *The Mind of the Soviet Fighting Man* (Westport, Conn.: Greenwood Press, 1984), pp. 43–45.
9. G. Avrutskiy and A. A. Neduva, *Treatment of the Mentally Ill* (Moscow: Meditsina, 1981), p. 6.
10. Ibid., p. 26.
11. Ibid., p. 424.

Bibliographic Essay

Although there is no major work on the subject of Soviet military psychiatry, several books and articles are available that offer genuine insights into the subject. One ought to be aware, however, that the Soviet regime has been engaged in a systematic effort to rewrite the official history of Soviet psychology at least since the 1950s and that it has made a constant effort since 1917 to produce works demonstrating that Soviet psychiatric theory and practice are consistent with Marxist-Leninist thought.

As a prelude to serious investigation into the subject of Soviet combat psychiatry, the researcher should at least become familiar with works that bear the characteristic marks of the regime's handiwork. Good examples of this effort are found in A. V. Barabanshchikov, K. K. Platonov, and N. F. Fedenko, "On the History of Soviet Military Psychology," *Soviet Psychology* (Fall 1968), pp. 48–56 and Mikhail Gourvetch's work, *A Textbook for Students of Psychiatry* (Moscow: Government Publishing House, 1948). Gourvetch's book is valuable not only as a textbook for basic instruction in psychiatry but also for its efforts to make its physiological premises square with Marxist theory. Probably the best example of the Soviet effort to rewrite the history of Soviet psychology is found in A. A. Smirnov, "Soviet Psychologists In Defense of the Motherland During the Great Patriotic War," *Journal of Soviet Psychiatry* (1975), pp. 13–30.

A very valuable source is *The Experience of the Soviet Medical Services During the Great Patriotic War*, published in Moscow in 1948. This encyclopedic compendium in several volumes was compiled by medical officers of the Red Army detailing the wartime experiences of all branches of the medical corps. One complete volume is devoted to psychiatric casualties and the manner in which the Soviets treated them. Unfortunately, this work is not available in the West. A copy is rumored to be in a medical library in East Germany, and access to it by foreigners in the Soviet Union is very carefully controlled.

Those fortunate enough to obtain access to Soviet medical libraries ought to investigate the *Korsakov Journal of Psychiatry and Neurology* published in Moscow. In the early 1950s, Dr. Abram Cvyadosch published pieces of his dissertation dealing with psychiatric casualties in World War II in article form in this journal. Although one has to hunt for the articles, they make interesting, if fragmentary, reading.

More easily available are a number of technical works published in translation by the Defense Technical Information Center at Cameron Station in Virginia. G. Avrutskiy and A. A. Neduva's work, *Treatment of the Mentally Ill* (Moscow: Meditsina Press, 1981), is a highly technical work that delineates treatment methodologies for the mentally ill, including drug therapies. Its primary value in terms of combat psychiatry rests in its discussion of affective and reactive states resulting from traumatic shock. Y. A. Aedsandrovskiy, *Tranquilizers and Psychostimulants for Patients with Borderline Neuropsychiatric Disorders* (Moscow: Meditsina Press, 1979) is also a good technical work valuable for its discussions of drug therapies available to Soviet psychiatrists.

A number of basic works deal with Soviet psychology/psychiatry expressed in terms of doctrine for conditioning the Soviet soldier to withstand the stress of battle. Among these are V. V. Shelyag, A. D. Glotochkin, and K. K. Platonov, eds., *Military Psychology: A Soviet View* (Moscow: Government Publishing House, 1972). This work is probably among the best known sources on the subject in the United States if only because it has been translated into English by the U.S. Air Force and has been made widely available through the Superintendent of Documents, U.S. Government Printing Office, Washington, D.C. It is useful only in a most general sense, however. Better works addressing the conditioning of the soldier are A. S. Zheltov, ed., *The Soldier and War: Problems in the Political, Morale and Psychological Training of the Soviet Serviceman* (Moscow: Ministry of Defense Publishing House, 1974), and L. Pavlovich and L. Grimak, *Psychological Training of the Parachutist* (Moscow: Military Publishing House, 1971).

Anyone interested in developing an accurate history of Soviet military psychiatry—or even a purely medical history of psychiatry and psychology—must put together such a history without the help of any major historical sources on the subject. It is particularly instructive, for example, that between 1914 and 1939 *The Lancet* did not publish a single article

Bibliographic Essay

on the subject of military psychiatry. The only source of information still resides with those individuals, Soviet psychiatrists and psychologists, who are still alive and either lived the history itself or were fortunate to have access to information provided by others who had lived the history. This book is one attempt to make a small inroad into a field whose boundaries have yet to be explored.

Index

abasia, 149
abreaction, 69
Academy of Pedagological Sciences, 16
acute shock, 143, 147
affective fear, 145–47
alcohol, 117
alcoholic neuropathy, 5
aloe, 69
aminazine, 147
amitriptylene, 146
Ananyev, Boris, 14
army level hospital, 57, 65–68, 127–28, 134–36
Asratyan, Ashraf, 31
asthasia, 149
auditory hallucinations, 146
Avrutsky, G. Y., 30
autogenic training, 140
autosuggestion, 117, 140
azaphine, 146

babamyl, 147
barbiturates, 68

battle discipline, Soviet, 114–16
battle fatigue, 144
battleshock, 50, 60, 65, 67, 68, 73, 74, 86, 87, 94, 119, 120, 131, 143
Bekhterev, Vladimir, 4, 7, 8, 21
Bekhterev Institute, 14, 17, 27, 28, 30, 31
benzodiazephine, 118
BGTO, 100
big psychiatry, 5, 51, 59
biological psychiatry, 5–6, 21, 37, 69, 77
biological shock, 133, 140
biological therapy, 139
blindness, 60, 67, 146
Bodalev, Alexei, 16
brain edema, 69
brain lesions, 60, 69
brain shock, 60
brom, 68
bruising of the brain, 60

caffeine, 117
calcium chloride, 69

calcium IV, 143
cardiac bromide, 143
chlorophonphysine, 147
chloryl hydrate, 68, 143
clinical psychotherapy, 142
combat medical doctrine, Soviet, 126
combat reaction, 50, 58–59, 153
commotion, 51, 53, 60
concussion, 51–52, 60, 67, 68, 131
conditioned reflex, 78–81, 102, 105, 108, 119
conditioned response, 83, 106, 145
confused states, 36
"consciousness as action," 30
contractive paralysis, 63
contusion, 51–52, 60, 67, 68, 131
conversion reactions, 61, 65, 67
conversion states, 63
conversion symptoms, 62
conversion syndrome, 61
convulsions, 67
coping, 76

Defense Intelligence Agency, 127
delirium of pursuit, 146
depressed psychogenic shock, 145
depression psychosis, 61
depressive reactions, 143–46
diencephalon, 77
dimedrol, 147
district level hospital, 127–28
division level hospital, 133–35
Donnelly, Christopher, 96, 97, 103
DOSAFF, 42, 96, 100, 125
draft avoidance, 124
draft commissariat, 122
"driven system", 116, 124
drug industry, Soviet, 116–20

Dupuy, T. R., 40
dynamic stereotype, 81, 115

edema, 60
electric stimulation, 40
electroconvulsive therapy, 63
emotion, 74; cortical emotions, 85; collapse, 84; emotional states, 84–85; exhaustion, 83; shock, 80; sub-cortical emotions, 85; theory of, 82–87; trauma, 50
epileptic stroke, 50
evacuation syndrome, 34
"evil" will, 80
excitement, 79
excitation, 81
exhaustion, 86, 118, 149
exogenic symptomatic psychosis, 149
extract of magnolia vine, 117
extreme psychomotor excitation, 147

failure to adapt, 42, 47, 121
fatigue, 94–95
fear, 84–85, 94–95
"fibs", 69
first signal system, 78–79
folk medicines, 68, 116
Freud, Sigmund, 3, 7, 12, 21, 69, 85, 91
front level hospital, 56–57, 65–68, 127–28, 134–36
fugue states, 36, 61, 63, 69

GABA, 118, 149
Gal, Reuven, 90
Germanic School, 4–8, 12
ginseng, 69
Glantz, Robert, 41, 44
goldroot, 69

Index

hallucinations, 149
herb medicine compounds, 68–69
heroism, 87, 90–91
higher nervous system, 77
hypnotherapy, 140
hypersthenic neurasthenia, 148
hyposthenic neurasthenia, 148
hysteria, 53, 61, 67; hysterical blindness, 36; hysterical excitement, 36; hysterical neurosis, 143, 149; hysterical psychosis, 143; hysterical stupor, 147

ICD–9, 123, 143
ilenium, 146
imbecillia, 42, 123
immunizing conditioning program, 94–96
individual replacement system, 66, 127
induction, 79
inhibition, 79, 81
innervation, 81
Institute of Forensic Psychiatry, 122–23
Institute of Higher Nervous Activity, 27, 31
Institute of Industrial Design, 27–28
Institute of Philosophy of the National Academy of Sciences, 16
Institute of Psychology of the Georgian Academy of Sciences, 14
Institute of Toxicology, 30–31

Kaufmann Method, 62–63
Khrushchev, Nikita, 18
Kirov Military Academy, 28–29, 39, 118
Komsomol, 100
Korsakoff, Sergei, 4–5
Korsakoff's psychosis, 4

Kraepelin, Emil, 4
Krilov, A. A., 31
Kuzmin, Ivgeny, 16

Lapin, I. P., 30
Leningrad Military District Hospital, 134
Leningrad School, 4
Leontiev, Alexei, 14, 16
lesions, 67
levopromazine, 147
librium, 118
local paralysis, 36
Lomov, Boris, 15, 16, 18, 28
Luria, A. R., 14–17

magnesium, 69
magnesium IV, 143
magnesium sulphate, 147
mailbox grants, 15
"malleability of the psyche," 75–76
"man-collective-military machine," 98
mandarin root, 69
Marlowe, David, 90, 104
Marshall, S. L. A., 91
Medical Commission of the Academy of Medical Sciences, 16
medical evacuation, 55–57
medical somatic approach, 5
medical treatment structure, Soviet, 130–32
melancholia, 85
melipramine, 146
Miasishchev, Vladimir, 4, 14, 17
microbleeding, 60
military training, Soviet, 104–9
MMPI, 20
moral combat training, 90
Moscow Clinic #5, 23
Moscow Institute of Psychology, 14

Moscow School, 4, 15
mutism, 60, 74

narcohypnosis, 69
narcopsychotherapy, 140
narrowing of consciousness, 89
nation in arms, 98–99
natrium bromide, 68
need satisfaction, 83
negative emotion, 83
neurasthenia, 36, 69, 143, 148
neuroleptics, 146–47
neurophysiological approach, 4
neuropsychiatric casualty rates, Soviet, 47; US, 47–48
New Red Legions, xi
new socialist man, 100
nicotine, 118
nonpsychogenic reactive states, 145
nootropes, 148
nosological biological psychiatry, 4–5

Octobrists, 99
oligaphrenia, 123
operant therapy, 23
Operation Little Saturn, 45
organic needs, 80
orienting response, 77–84, 89, 94, 95, 104, 115
orthogenic training, 23
orthonomic reactions, 77

pain, 94–95
panic, 82–85, 95
pantacrene, 143
paralysis, 60–63, 67, 82, 74, 146
partial narrowing of consciousness, 86
Pavlov, Ivan, 4, 9–10, 21, 76–77, 88–89, 94–95, 104, 106
penal battalion, 52–56, 114

pentatine, 118
perphenazine, 146
People's Commissariat for the Defense of the USSR, 39
People's Commissariat of Public Health, 142
"pharmacological era of psychiatry," 139
Pharmacological Laboratory of the Psycho-Neurological Research Institute, 27–30
phenamine, 118
phenaput, 118
phenazapen, 146
Pioneers, 99
Plantanov, Konstantine, 16
pokey drill, 105
Political Academy, 16, 137
political officer, 16, 51–59, 115, 127, 138
post-traumatic stress disorder, 55
powdered reindeer horn, 69
preventive psychiatry, 142
primary signal system, 80
principle of expectancy, 52, 67, 71, 133
principle of immediacy, 54, 71
principle of proximity, 35, 37, 52, 71
principle of reflection, 77–78
psychasthenia, 149
psychiatric triage, 135
psychiatric screening, 121–26, 131
psychiatric treatment, 139–50
psychic tension, 79, 81, 89
psychogenic analysis, 8
psychogenic stupor, 146
psychoprisons, 142
psychostimulators, 94, 117–19, 147, 149
psychotrophic drugs, 140–41
"pull" system, 112

Index

"push" system, 112
pyrazdol, 146

radiation, 79
rational psychiatry, 75
rational psychotherapy, 140
reactive delirious psychosis, 143–46
reactive psychosis, 68, 146–49, 153
reactive states, 143–46
Red Professors, 8
reflexive conditioning, 102
reflex theory of the psyche, 4, 76–77
reflexology, 77
replacement depot, 128, 134
Russian Red Cross Society, 34
Russo-Japanese War, 34, 35, 36, 39, 54

scar tissue, 69
schizophasia, 67
Schlovsky, Victor, 17
Sechenev, I. M., 76
second signal system, 9, 21, 78, 79, 80–88, 91, 92, 145
secondary gain, 36, 131, 145
seizures, 68
"self-help for the soldier," 129–30
sensory delirium, 147
"sick book riders," 124
siduzium, 146
Simoniov, Pavel, 31
simplistic battle drills, 109
small psychiatry, 6, 50, 51, 56, 59, 61, 71, 127, 135, 148
social conditioning, 97–101, 102
socialist man, 75, 94
socio-rehabilitative therapy, 139
sodium bromide, 68
Solobyov, Uri, 29
Soyuz, 119

special psychiatric teams, 136
Speech Therapy Center of the Moscow Health District, 17
Spivak, Leonid, 28, 118
Stalin, Josef, 7, 8, 13, 39, 140
"steeling the will," 19, 116
stupor, 69
suggestion in a state of wakefullness, 140
suicide, 138
Sullivan, H. S., 8
surdomutism, 36, 53, 61, 63, 67, 147
symptomatic psychosis, 143
syndocarb, 118, 147

temperament, 81
Teplov, Boris, 14
terror, 13, 84, 87
therapy, types of; electro convulsive, 139; insular comotose, 139; medical convulsive, 139; narcotic sleep, 139; traumatic, 145–48
ticket out, 53, 67
tightened reactive state, 146
Timofeev, Nicolai, 28
torpor, 85
triftazin, 146
trioxizine, 118
trisedil, 146
tranquilizers, 94, 117, 118, 149
trauma induced psychosis, 145
traumatic encephalopathy, 60
tryphotizine, 147
twilight states, 149

udar, 50
unconscious, Soviet view of, 76–77
unit replacement system, 66, 127

Valaam, 70
valeriana, 69, 143
valium, 118
vegeostabilizer, 148
VNITTE, 27–28
volitional strength, 80–87, 95

war tremors, 152
water therapy, 40

Wexler intelligence scale, 20
will, 80–81

Yarmolenka, Augusta, 14

zone of excitement, 78–79
"Zaranitza," 99–100
Zeigarnick, Bluma, 14

About the Author

RICHARD A. GABRIEL is Professor of Politics at St. Anselm College in Manchester, New Hampshire. He is a former army intelligence officer and reserve major assigned to the Pentagon. A consultant to the House and Senate Armed Services Committees, he is the author of fifteen books and scores of articles on military subjects. Among his books are a number of definitive works, including *Crisis in Command, The New Red Legions* (2 vols., Greenwood Press, 1980) and *The Mind of the Soviet Fighting Man* (Greenwood Press, 1984), *To Serve With Honor* (Greenwood Press, 1982), and *Fighting Armies* (3 vols., Greenwood Press, 1983). His most recent work is *Military Incompetence: Why The American Military Doesn't Win.*

Dr. Gabriel has held academic posts at the Brookings Institution and the Army Intelligence School, and at Hebrew University in Jerusalem. He is currently a fellow at the Department of Combat Psychiatry at the Walter Reed Army Institute of Research and the Center for the Study of Intelligence in Washington, D.C.

Recent Titles in
Contributions in Military Studies

History of the Art of War: Within the Framework of Political History, The Modern Era
Hans Delbrück, translated by Walter J. Renfroe, Jr.

In Peace and War: Interpretations of American Naval History, 1775–1984. A Second Edition
Edited by Kenneth J. Hagan

America's Forgotten Wars: The Counterrevolutionary Past and Lessons for the Future
Sam C. Sarkesian

The Heights of Courage: A Tank Leader's War on the Golan
Avigdor Kahalani

The Tainted War: Culture and Identity in Vietnam War Narratives
Lloyd B. Lewis

Shaping a Maritime Empire: The Commercial and Diplomatic Role of the American Navy, 1829–1861
John H. Schroeder

The American Occupation of Austria: Planning and Early Years
Donald R. Whitnah and Edgar L. Erickson

Crusade in Nuremberg: Military Occupation, 1945–1949
Boyd L. Dastrup

The Dogma of the Battle of Annihilation: The Theories of Clausewitz and Schlieffen and Their Impact on the German Conduct of Two World Wars
Jehuda L. Wallach

Jailed for Peace: The History of American Draft Law Violators, 1658–1985
Stephen M. Kohn

Against All Enemies: Interpretations of American Military History from Colonial Times to the Present
Kenneth J. Hagan and William R. Roberts

Citizen Sailors in a Changing Society: Policy Issues for Manning the United States Naval Reserve
Edited by Louis A. Zurcher, Milton L. Boykin, and Hardy L. Merritt

Strategic Nuclear War: What the Superpowers Target and Why
William C. Martel and Paul L. Savage